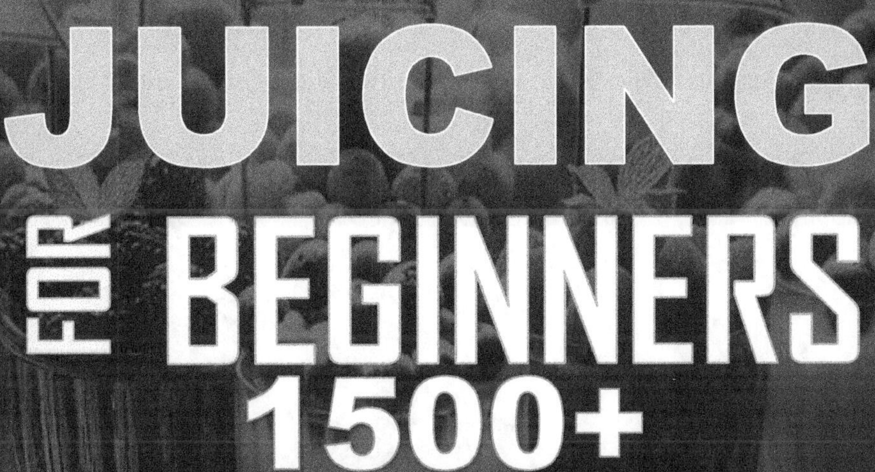

JUICING FOR BEGINNERS

1500+

Days of Vibrant Juicing with Easy and Effortless

Recipes to Lose Weight, Gain Energy, Detox,

Longevity, Smooth Skin and 7-Days Meal Plan

PAULA J. EVANS

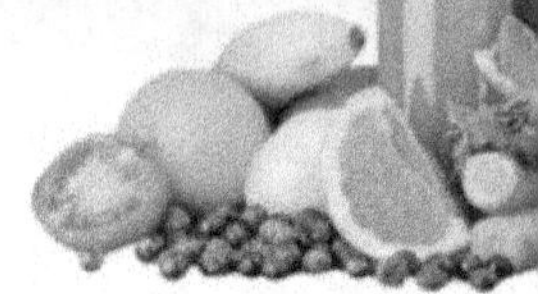

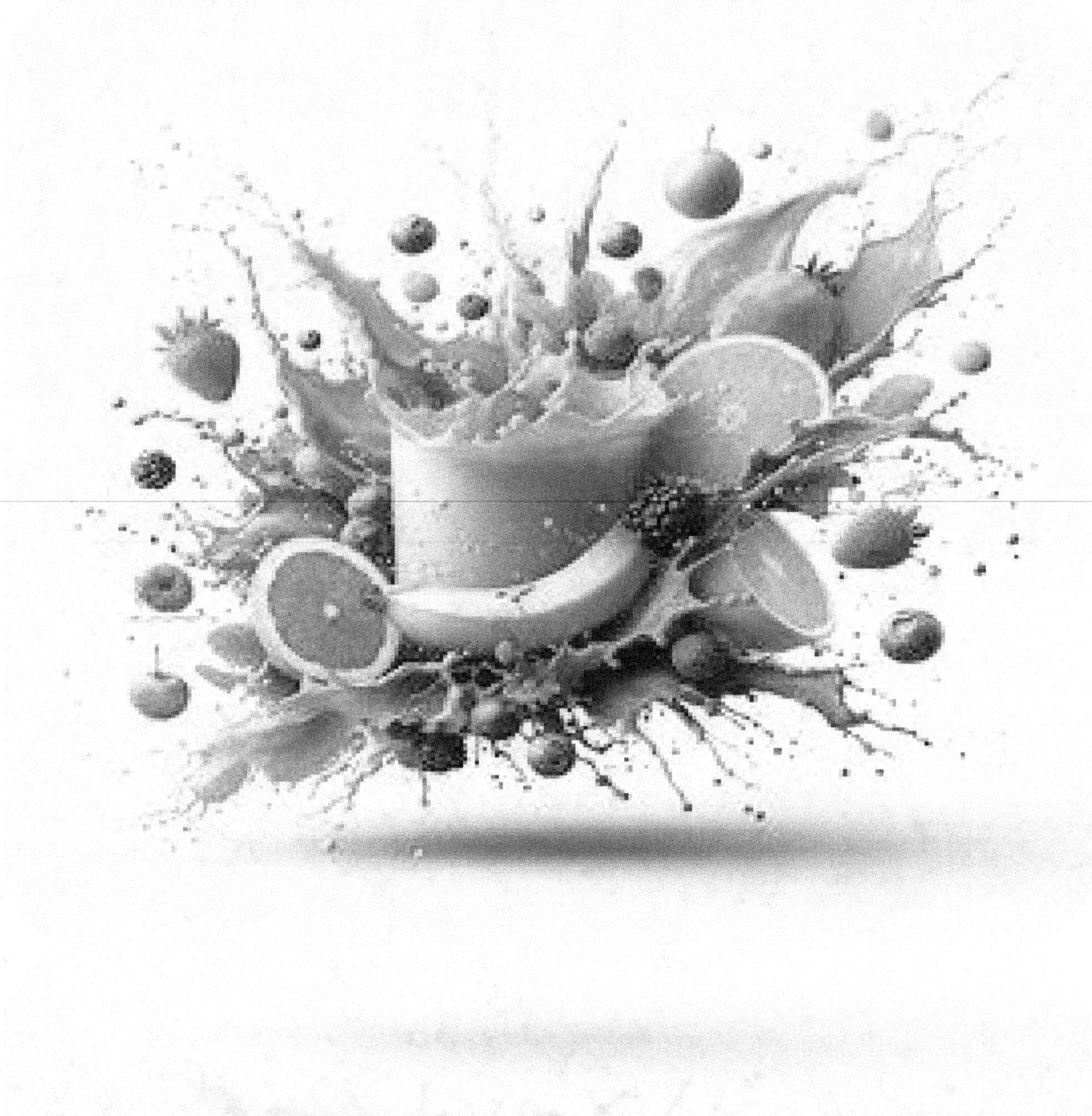

TABLE OF CONTENTS

INTRODUCTION

Tired of feeling sluggish? Juice your way to "Hallelujah!" with Juicing for Beginners!

This isn't your mama's juicing guide. Ditch the jargon and grab your blender, cause we're making juicing easy, fun, and totally beginner-friendly.

Think glowing skin, explosive energy, and a happier gut party – all within reach of a delicious green concoction.

<u>Inside, you'll find:</u>

<u>100</u>+ **crave-worthy recipes:** No kale-flavored tears here! Think tropical twists, creamy wonders, and flavor bombs to rock your taste buds.

Simple steps, zero stress: We break it down from choosing a juicer to mastering the art of the blend (no science degree required!).

Science-backed benefits: Feel good knowing you're not just sipping sugar water – discover the real health magic of juicing. ✦

Bonus! We don't stop at recipes. Find tips, tricks, to keep you juicing like a pro and more

Ready to ditch the fatigue and say "Hallelujah!" to a healthier you? Scroll up, grab your copy, and let's get juicing!

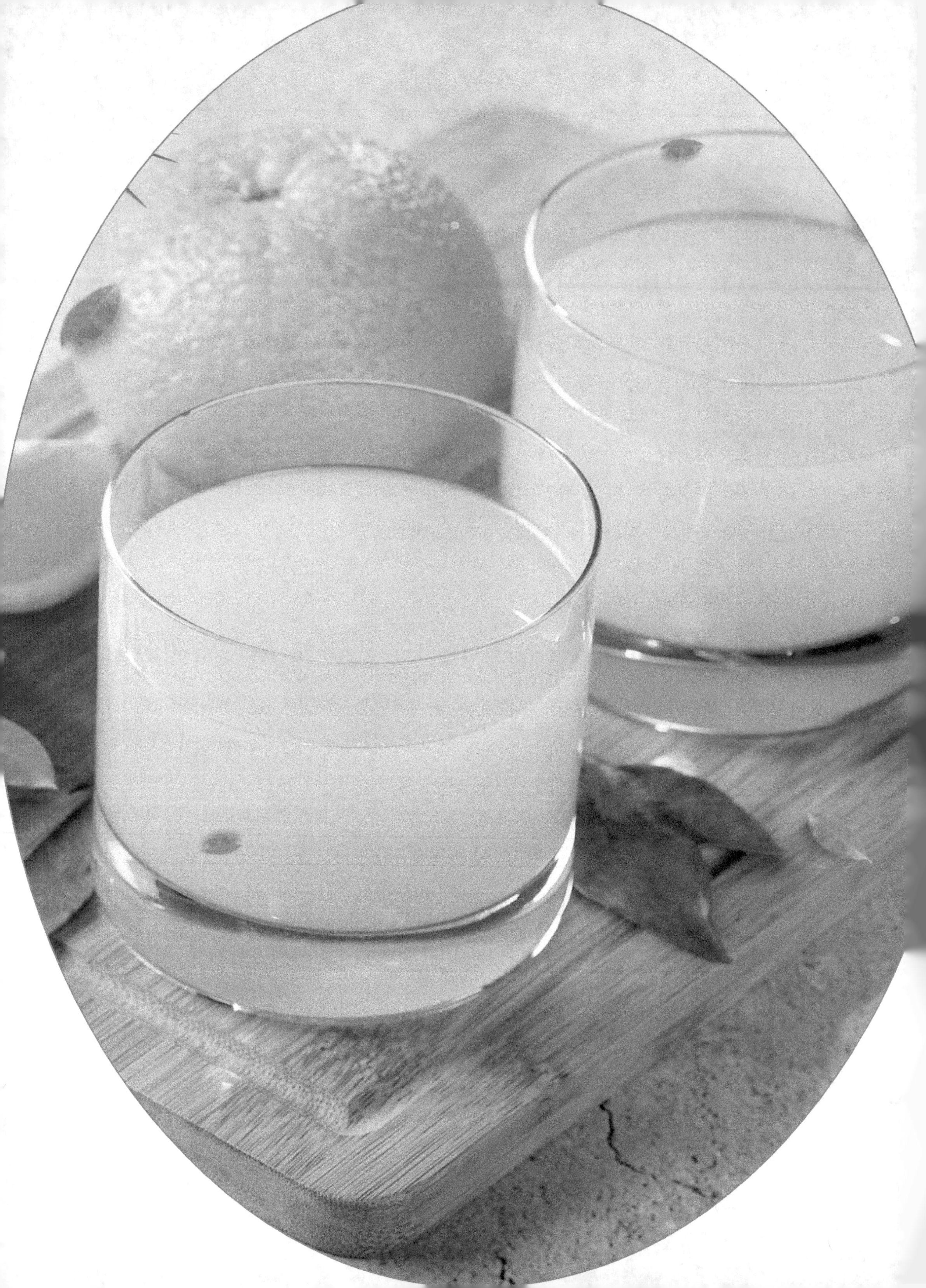

How Does Juicing Work?

Simply explained, the process of extracting juice from fruits and vegetables is referred to as juicing, using a citrus press, juicing may be done manually, or it can be done using a machine performed with the help of a juicer, which is a kind of electric home device. Generally speaking, the term "juicing" refers to the process of boosting your consumption of natural juices. consuming freshly squeezed juices of fruits and vegetables on a regular basis to meet your daily recommended consumption.

There are many different reasons why people juice, the most of them are linked to their health. In addition to improving your intake of essential nutrients, juicing also delivers advantages for weight reduction, cleansing, and more.

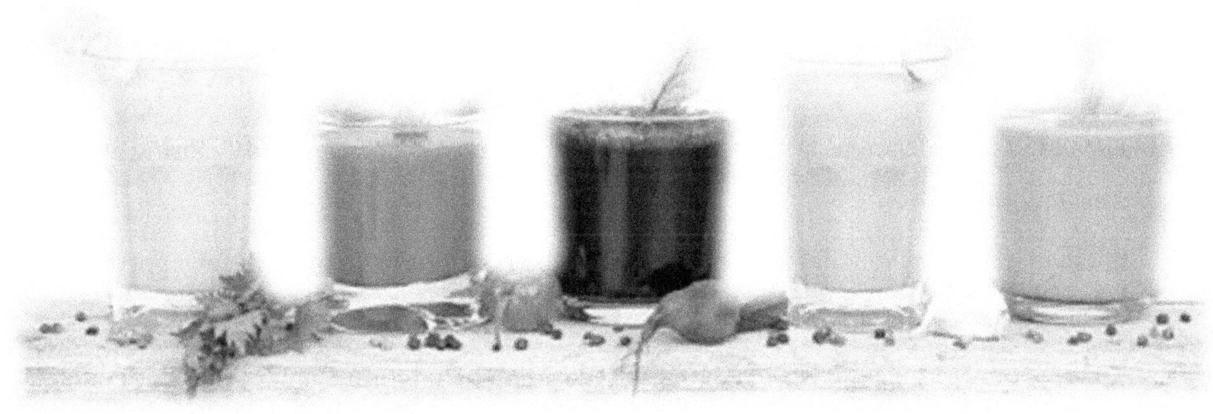

Benefits of Juicing Versus Eating Raw Fruits and Vegetables

Registered dieticians and other health-care professionals are split on the problem of whether or not juicing is more healthful than eating raw fruits and vegetables. While juicing obviously isn't harmful, there is some controversy whether on if it is healthier than simply eating the fruits and veggies themselves. Jennifer K. Nelson, a licensed dietitian, says that "juicing extracts the juice from fresh fruits or vegetables. the resultant liquid includes most of the vitamins, minerals, and plant compounds (phytonutrients) contained in the entire fruit." As many detractors of the juicing trend are eager to point out, however, a major chunk of the fiber content of fruits and vegetables is lost during the juicing process.

In order to grasp the differences between juicing and eating raw fruits and vegetables, you need to grasp the fundamentals of how a juicer works. A juicer is a kitchen device that takes the labor out of extracting the juice from fresh fruits and vegetables. These gadgets are motor operated, and they come in a range of sizes. Though the mechanics of various models may vary, finest juicers demand you to force the fresh fruits and veggies using a feed tube. Inside, the equipment extracts the juice from the plant fibers, sifting off the seeds, skin, and pulp. The fresh juice then leaves the machine by a spout and into the selected glass or container.

For many individuals, making use of a juicer is a fast and simple approach to enhance the daily consumption of fruits and vegetables. While it is true that some of the fiber content of the raw fruits and vegetables is lost during juicing, there are several specific advantages that juicing gives over consuming raw fruits and vegetables. These include:

- Juicing is a wonderful option if you do not generally enjoy eating uncooked fruits and veggies.
- The results are delicious—you can even mask the flavor of veggies by pairing them with your favorite fruits.
- Juicing is a fast and uncomplicated operation; the resultant juice may be consumed with you for an on-the-go supper.
- Adding some of the pulp to your squeezed juice can help return some of its fiber content.
- Juicing does not need you to peel or cut the vegetables prior utilizing it (depending on the kind of juicer you purchase).
- Homemade juices have a fresh-squeezed flavor; store-bought juices just can't compare.
- Juicing is an excellent technique to help your kids obtain the vitamins and minerals.
- Leftover pulp from juicing may be utilized in baked items, such as muffins, or as a foundation for homemade stocks and broths.
- Juicing is an affordable approach to make use of fruits and vegetables that are about to spoil.

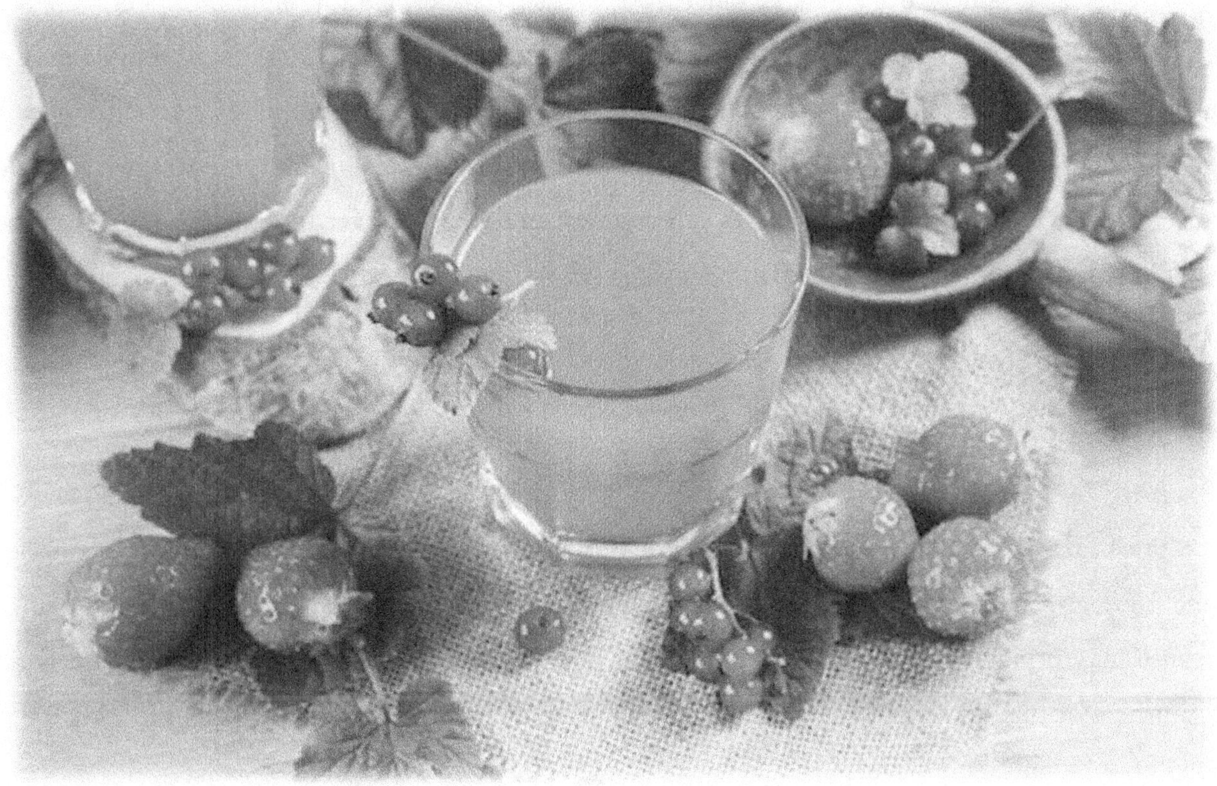

While the procedure of juicing is as basic as feeding fresh fruits and veggies through your juicer, there are a few things you may need to do before you take the initial step. You do not need to bother about peeling or cutting your vegetables, but you should take the time to wash it beforehand. Even if you purchasing organic food, it might still have germs. Once you've carefully wash the produce, you need to prepare your juicer. These preparations will vary based on the kind of juicer. If your juicer has a pulp basket or canister, lining it with a plastic bag will make cleaning simpler.

Next, set the juicer on and feed the vegetables through it on the speed suggested in the manufacturer's instructions. Remember, you don't always need to peel or slice the vegetables, but you may need to cut it in half or rip huge leaves into tiny pieces for them to fit into the feed tube.

Refer to the guidelines given with your juicer to find the appropriate speed for various sorts of vegetables. (Softer items like berries may need a moderate speed whereas tougher vegetables like as beets or apples may demand a greater speed.) After you finish passing the vegetables through the juicer, check the pulp basket or canister. If you encounter bits of unprocessed food, or if the pulp is still moist, pass it through the machine again to extract as much juice as possible.

Once you've done, you may enjoy your tasty beverage. It is vital to consume your juice as soon as possible after pressing it because, like other fresh foods exposed to air, it might grow germs if you let it sit for too long. If you generate more juice than you can swallow at one time, keep the excess in an airtight jar in the refrigerator for up to forty-eight hours. Glass containers are better since plastic may contain BPA (bisphenol A), a substance that may cause major health concerns. If you do preserve your juice, fill the container as full as you can manage—over time, extra oxygen in the container may diminish the nutrients in your juice.

Juicing for Detoxification

If you are aware with the juicing movement, you may have also heard of a juice detox. Also known as a juice fast, it includes drinking nothing but fruit and vegetable liquids for a certain amount of time. Though lengthy term fasting of this type is normally not suggested, a three- to five-day juice cleanse may bring several health advantages. Sceptics of juice cleansing indicate that there is no scientific evidence to support the belief that eating fresh fruit and vegetable juices can clear your body of pollutants.

While juicing may not be a miracle cure to the world's health difficulties, it does have a variety of advantages that may help to cleanse and cleanse your body. The current Western diet is centered on processed foods, which comprise filled with artificial preservatives, flavors, and other poisons. Thankfully, the human body is built to filter out and remove these poisons; yet, the usual Western diet delivers a hazardous burden far greater than the body is capable of managing. Your liver, kidneys, lungs, and skin are the major detoxification organs in your body, and when they become overwhelmed, your body may begin collecting surplus toxins in your fat cells and tissues. Over time, your body will become toxic and you may suffer a range of undesirable side effects, including indigestion, allergies, constipation, dry hair and skin, acne, and more.

It is crucial to note that fresh fruit and vegetable juices will not miraculously make the poisons in your body gone. Juicing can, nonetheless, play a part in naturally detoxing your body. Engaging in a juice detox implies that you will quit harming your body with toxic-laden manufactured meals, substituting them instead with nutrient-rich liquids. If, after you finish your juice cleanse, you continue to avoid processed foods when develop a habit of ingesting fresh fruits and vegetables, your body will naturally begin to recuperate from its toxic overburden. By decreasing your intake of pollutants, your body will be able to concentrate on stored toxins and eliminate them from your system, which will result in enhanced overall health.

Choosing a Juicer

Choosing a juicer might be a complicated procedure if you don't comprehend the fundamentals. Before you start shopping for your new juicer, take the time to read about the three main sorts so you can choose whether selection is best for you.

The three basic kinds of juicers are: centrifugal juicers, masticating juicers, and triturating juicers, each kind has its own list various positives and downsides, thus in order to find the correct one for your case, you need to think about what characteristics you desire. You should also pick what price range you are prepared to explore, since juicers may be fairly expensive.

Centrifugal Juicers

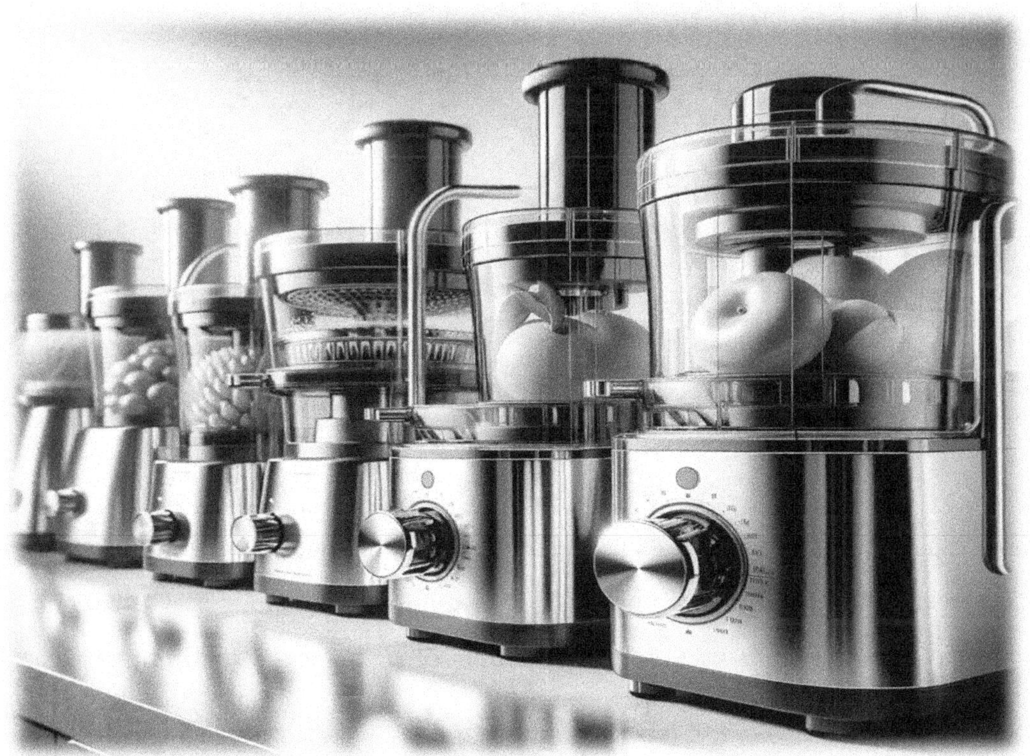

A centrifugal juicer is possibly the simplest sort of juicer. For one thing, it is simple to use and easy to clean. Also, these juicers employ grated basket that functions as a rotating blade, grinding the vegetables and extracting the juice. The pulp stays in the basket while the liquid goes through the apertures and exits the appliance via the spout. These juicers operate really rapidly and are one of the most economical solutions, but they are not adequately adapted to handle exceptionally hard crops or pitted fruits.

Masticating Juicers

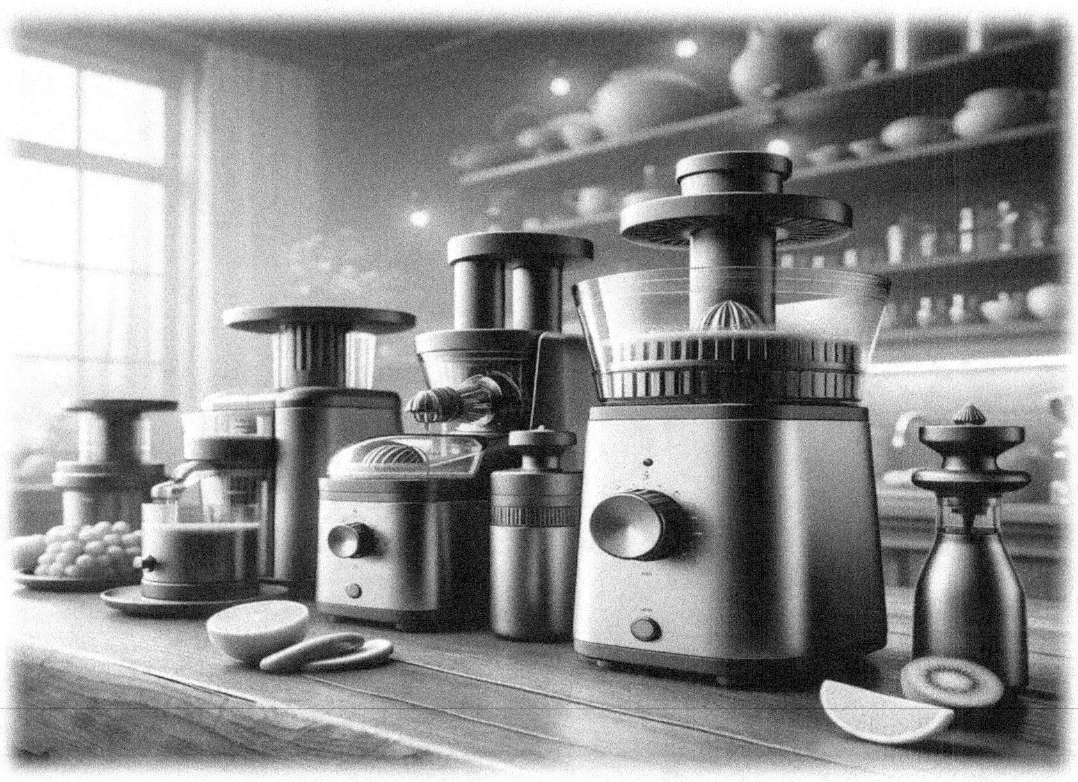

A masticating juicer runs more slowly than a centrifugal juicer. These juicers function by kneading and grinding the material in the feed chute, squeezing the juice out into a container. The advantage of this sort of juicer is because it runs at a slower pace than other juicers, which implies that it generates less heat. Because the juicer doesn't become particularly hot, fewer enzymes are destroyed, thus the juice should not oxidise too much, giving it a longer shelf life.

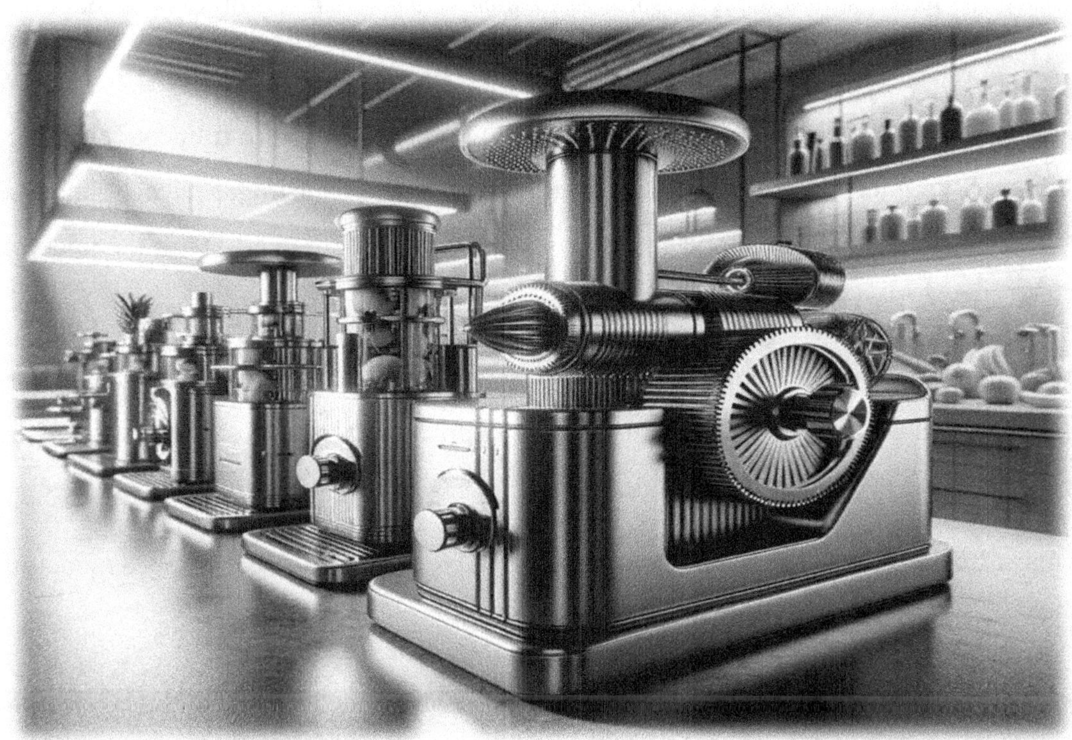

A triturating juicer is a twin-gear juicer that employs a two-step juicing process. When fruit is put through the juicer, it is first pulverized and then it is pushed. These appliances may be a bit expensive, but they are the most efficient. They also emit less heat, which is good for keeping enzymes and limiting oxidization.

Essential Tips in Selecting a Great Juicer

So, you now know how good juicing is for your health. You are currently intending to acquire a juicer for your requirements. Before purchasing a juicer, you must realize that not all juicers are the same. There are various changes and you should choose for the one that matches your requirements best.

Here are some suggestions for picking a fantastic juicer:

- ❖ The juicer should be able to juice all fruits and vegetables. Therefore, it should be a citrus and centrifugal juicer and have masticating qualities.
- ❖ It should be simple to use and clean.

- ❖ The juice that is separated should be of great quality.
- ❖ Finally, the juicer should meet your budget. Determine how often you will use the juicer and then purchase appropriately.

Masticating juicers have been determined to be the best. They "chew" the entire fruits or vegetables and are known to create juices with better nutritional content than a centrifugal juicer. The juice generated by these juicers contains less oxygen and, consequently, extends shelf life of the juice.

Certain masticating juicers feature a single cutter, while others have double gears. They employ two gears of cylindrical form that fit together firmly, smashing the fruits or veggies. Nutritionists typically suggest the twin gear juicer. But, cleaning is a long procedure with these juicers, since the distance between the gears is quite little.

These juicers may also do extra duties. All of them are dependable since they use low speed induction motors.

The third form of masticating juicer is the single auger juicer that is low speed but still juices rapidly. They can also juice wheatgrass. Centrifugal juicers, on the other hand, feature a flat cutting blade with a basket, as opposed to the steel teeth on the masticating juicer's cutter.

In today's world, individuals live a fast-paced existence. Not many individuals have the time to stop and inspect their body. You run about, go to work, meet clients, exercise, sleep less than your body requires, and consume junk food, perhaps too much. Such a life requires an injection of health regularly. It requires a regular dose of juicing. So, how does juicing work? Is it healthy or unhealthy? The solution to these questions are depending on the method juice is ingested and the meals that the juice replaces.

Whole fruits and vegetables include fiber that is lost in juicing. For example, compare a full apple with apple juice. It can be observed that apple juice has no detectable level of fiber. Additionally, roughly 4 apples are needed for creating 1 cup of apple juice, depending on the juiciness and size of apples. Each apple contains around 3.5 grams of dietary fiber, which is a total of 12 to 14 grams of dietary fiber of 4 apples. These 14 grams of fiber are lost in the cup of apple juice. How much more healthful the juice would be if the fiber could be added to the diet!

Consider the difference in digestion of a whole vegetable or fruit and liquid meal, which is the juice. Juices are really processed food. Resultantly, nutrients and sugar are released significantly more rapidly in the body. It is easier to drink juice of more fruits than to eat that amount of fruits or vegetables. vegetables. Therefore, juicing promotes fruit and vegetable consumption in the type of juices.

In addition to this, the body takes half an hour to digest the complete meal, whilst juices are instantly absorbed. Consequently, nutrients and sugars are released promptly and the body receives a fast burst of energy. But, despite the fact that fluids are more readily absorbed, the reality remains that the body loses the dietary fiber in liquids.

Benefits of Juicing

Here are the top advantages of juicing:

- Easy Assimilation - Since liquids don't contain fiber, the body quickly absorbs them. They bypass the process of digestion and reach the cells in less than 30 minutes. Your body receives a respite from the digestion process, providing it increased energy for cleaning, detoxing, and physical exertion.
- Better Absorption of Nutrients - Juices are excellent for you if your digestive system is weak. If you suffer from illnesses such as ulcers, reflux and others, the nutrients from your diet flow out. Juices absorb nutrition.
- Alkalinity - Juicing offers your body an alkaline environment, enhancing the immune system and raising energy, while lowering irritation and discomfort.
- Hydration Juicing hydrates your bodily cells, enhancing cell performance. Fresh fruit and vegetable juice supplies the water content that your body needs at the same time, juices also include minerals, vitamins, phytochemicals, and enzymes that are vital for your health.
- Micro-nutrients Maintenance – Cooking and preparing food modifies micro-nutrients, making it difficult for the body to absorb them. Juicing retains the micro-nutrients.
- Detoxification - Juicing is an efficient approach to cleanse your body. It cleanses the colon and digestive system, boosting the metabolism of the body.
- Chlorophyll - Plants contain chlorophyll, which has a distinctive structure. It augments the body's hemoglobin production capabilities; therefore, enhancing oxygen supply to the cells. This offers the body extra energy.

- Antioxidants Fruits and vegetables contain antioxidants that combat damaging free radicals. This slows down cell damage, thereby slowing down age or susceptibility to cancer.

- Healing powers - Fruits and vegetables possess healing powers. You may build a unique prescription for a certain bodily requirement by method of juicing. This increases immunity, strengthening bones, and boosting energy. When you can mix meals, your body is able to absorb the nutrients that aid healing.

- Volume - You are able to eat huge amounts of veggies and fruits that you would ordinarily not consume. Your body absorbs vital nutrients that are needed for optimal health. Juices have a high proportion of enzymes, minerals, and vitamins. Since these nutrients enter your bloodstream rapidly, your body receives the advantages immediately.

The Difference between Juice and Smoothies

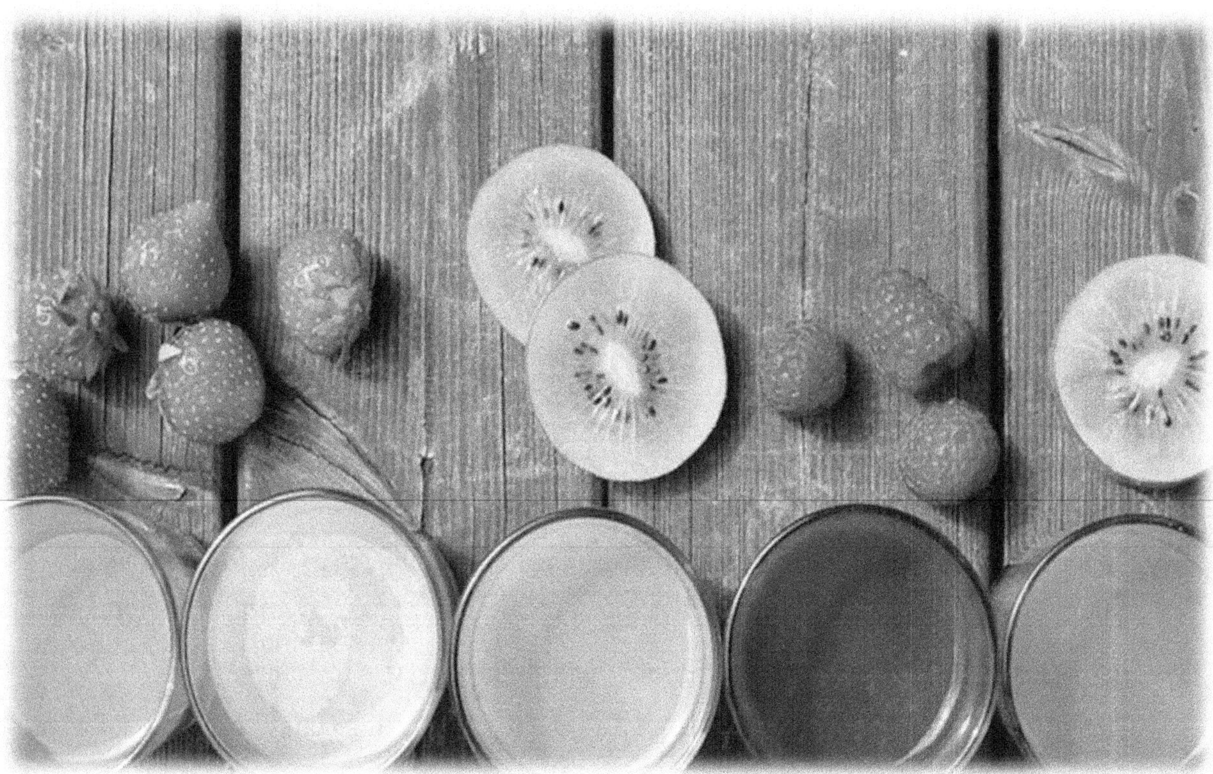

Both smoothies and juices include all of the key elements found in entire fruits and veggies. However, there are some distinctions between them, as stated below:

- Smoothies - Smoothies are created from entire fruits and vegetables. They are generated using a blender. Using entire fruits produces a full smoothie, making it equivalent to a full meal. A blender is used to prepare a smoothie.
- Smoothies have all the fiber that is found in whole meals and your digestive system gets a solid workout.
- Juicing - Juicing is the procedure in which the pulp and juice is separated using a juicer. The resulting juice is a thin liquid juice that is packed of nutrients. It is not extremely filling but moisturizes the body.

Fruits needed for healthy juice recipes:

- Apple
- Avocado
- Banana
- Blackberry
- Black cherry
- Blood orange
- Blueberry
- Cantaloupe
- Grape
- Grapefruit
- Kiwi
- Lemon
- Lime
- Mango
- Melon
- Orange
- Papaya
- Passion fruit
- Peach
- Pear
- Pineapple
- Pomegranate
- Raspberry
- Strawberry
- Tangerine

Health Benefits of Fruits

- **Apple:** Apples contain an antioxidant called quercetin, which helps to lower LDL (bad) cholesterol levels. These fruits are also rich in a soluble fiber called pectin, which may help eliminate dangerous heavy metals from the body.
- **Avocado:** Avocados are a fantastic source of heart-healthy fats (monounsaturated fats). In addition, avocados include potassium to control blood pressure, vitamin K to support bone health, and plant based protein.

- **Banana:** Bananas are rich in B vitamins, which assist support healthy sleep habits and minimize mood swings and irritation. This fruit also contains lots of vitamin C in addition to potassium and magnesium, all of which help to restore the body's supply of electrolytes. Bananas are inherently sweet—they may be pureed and incorporated into any of your favorite juices.

- **Blackberry:** In addition to being a good source of vitamin C, blackberries have significant quantities of calcium, potassium, iron, and fiber Berries like blackberries contain the greatest quantities of antioxidants of any fruit.

- **Black Cherry:** Cherries are a rich source of iron, which aids the body produce healthy blood cells. These fruits also contain an anti-carcinogenic molecule called ellagic acid, and contain high quantities of vitamins A and C. In addition to these nutrients, cherries also include antioxidant, anti-inflammatory, and antibacterial activities.

- **Orange:** Blood oranges are a kind of orange recognized for its crimson-colored flesh. This unusual hue is due to high quantities of anthocyanin, a kind of antioxidant pigment—their presence causes blood oranges higher in antioxidants than other oranges. Blood oranges are also a rich source of dietary fiber, vitamin C, calcium, and folate.

- **Blueberry:** Like apples, blueberries contain pectin as well as flavonoids, which may help lessen your risk for type 2 diabetes.

- Blueberries are particularly rich in vitamin C, potassium, and tannins, which have antiviral and antibacterial characteristics. Additionally, blueberries contain manganese, which assists to good bone formation.

- **Cantaloupe:** Cantaloupes are spherical melons with a brilliant orange flesh it is loaded with nutrients. Though rich of juice and sweet taste, melon is minimal in calories, and a great source of folic acid, beta carotene, fiber, potassium, and vitamin C. Unlike many fruits and veggies, cantaloupe also includes complex B vitamins.

- **Grape:** Grapes are rich in a variety of vitamins, including A, B, and C, in addition to minerals such as calcium, iron, phosphorus, magnesium, potassium, and selenium. Grapes also contain flavonoids, a potent antioxidant that can help repair damage caused by free radicals—this characteristic makes grapes a superb anti-aging aid.

- **Grapefruit:** Like other citrus fruits, grapefruit is a rich source of vitamin C. Grapefruit also includes limonene, a chemical that may aid lessen the risk of breast cancer. Additionally, grapefruits are a wonderful source of soluble fiber, which may help decrease harmful blood cholesterol levels.

- **Kiwi:** Kiwi is a fantastic source of vitamin C, which helps to cure wounds and maintain your teeth and gums healthy. These fruits also include vitamin K, vitamin E, folate, copper, and potassium. The enzymes discovered in kiwi have been demonstrated to relieve stomach troubles and may lower the look of wrinkles.

- **Lemon:** Lemon is generally said to be the most potent fruit for detoxification. It has been related to cancer prevention, relief from digestive difficulties, and lower risk for heart disease and stroke. Lemons are rich in calcium, magnesium, potassium, and phosphorus.

- **Lime:** Limes are very similar to lemons in their nutritional characteristics. These fruits are an excellent source of vitamin C, vitamin B6, folate, and potassium. Limes also contain flavonoids, a potent antioxidant, and numerous other phytonutrients.

- **Mango:** Mangoes contain both vitamin A and vitamin C, which produce them highly useful for boosting the immune system. Mangoes are an excellent supply of potassium, which has been demonstrated to control heart rate and blood pressure. They have also been related to lower risk for certain forms of cancer.

- **Melon:** Melons, such as honeydew and watermelon, possess both antioxidant and anti-cancer properties. These fruits contain adenosine, a naturally occurring substance that may lessen the risk for cancer and stroke.

- **Orange:** Oranges are recognized for their vitamin C concentration; however, they really contain more than 170 distinct phytonutrients. These fruits have been found to help shrink tumors, avoid blood clots, and decrease inflammation.

- **Papaya:** Papayas are recognized for its antioxidant and anti-cancer properties. These fruits contain powerful enzymes that assist to decrease constipation and support healthy digestion. Additionally, papayas are a rich source of potassium and vitamins A and C.

- **Fruit:** Passion fruit is an extremely fragrant fruit with a distinctive flavor. They are a rich source of nutritional fiber, vitamin A, vitamin C, and beta-carotene. Passion fruit is particularly high in potassium, which may aid manage blood pressure and lower the risk for cardiovascular disease.

- **Peach:** In addition to its delicious taste, peaches are also noted for being a good source of both vitamins A and potassium. These fruits also include boron and niacin, or vitamin B3, which has been demonstrated to minimize the risk for cardiovascular disease.

- **Pear:** Pears are a rich source of dietary fiber, vitamin C, boron, and potassium. These fruits have been utilized for a range of advantages, including as a diuretic, a cleaner, and a digestive aid.

- **Pineapple**: Pineapples are a wonderful source of iron, potassium, and vitamin C. These fruits also contain bromelain and other anti-inflammatory chemicals, which aid to enhance joint health. Pineapple has also been used as a natural diuretic and a mild laxative.

- **Pomegranate:** Pomegranates are a fantastic fruit for detoxifying and detoxifying the body. These fruits include vitamin C, magnesium, potassium, and beta-carotene—they have also been recognized as the third-highest fruit source of antioxidants. Pomegranates include lycopene and other phytonutrients that may help lessen the risk for prostate cancer.

- **Raspberry:** In addition to being high in vitamins C, K, and E, raspberries also include folate, manganese, copper, and iron. Raspberries have been found to help decrease LDL (bad) cholesterol and to block the development of some malignancies.

- **Strawberry:** Like other berries, strawberries are an excellent source of vitamin C, which helps to heal wounds and enhance gum and tooth health. Strawberries are also recognized to be antiviral, antioxidant, and anti-cancer properties. These berries have also been associated to reducing LDL (bad) cholesterol, reducing colon cancer, and guarding against Alzheimer's disease.

- **Tangerine:** Tangerines are an excellent source of calcium, copper, magnesium, potassium, and beta-carotene. These fruits also contain sulfur; this aids enhance detoxification of the liver. Additionally, tangerines have been demonstrated to have antibacterial, anti-cancer, diuretic, and decongestant qualities.

Vegetables needed for healthy juice recipes:

- Arugula
- Asparagus
- Beet
- Bell Pepper
- Bok Choy
- Broccoli
- Brussels Sprout
- Cabbage
- Carrot
- Cauliflower
- Celery
- Cilantro
- Collard Greens
- Cucumber

- Dandelion Greens
- Fennel
- Garlic
- Ginger
- Kale
- Mint
- Parsley
- Parsnip
- Pumpkin
- Romaine Lettuce
- Spinach
- Summer Squash
- Sweet Potato
- Swiss Chard
- Tomato
- Zucchini

Health Benefits of Vegetables

Arugula: Arugula is a lush green and a cruciferous vegetable, which says that it is rich in antioxidants and flavonoids that may help decrease your risk for cancer. Arugula is also a strong source for vitamins A, C, and K and a range of vital minerals.

Asparagus: Asparagus is a rich source of folate, which is necessary for fetal development. This veggie is also filled with antioxidants, they have been shown to minimize the look of aging and to delay cognitive deterioration. Asparagus also includes dietary fiber, chromium, and vitamins A, C, E, and K.

Beet: Beets and beet greens are a rich source of iron, choline, iodine, manganese, potassium, and vitamins A and C. Additionally, studies research demonstrated that beets assist to oxygenate the blood, improving performance when exercising.

Bell Pepper: Red, green, and yellow bell peppers have high quantities of vitamin C, which is vital for healing wounds and for preserving eye and gum health. They also contain vitamin A, which is a crucial component to skin and eye health.

Bok Choy: A kind of leafy Chinese cabbage, bok choy is rich in a diversity of phytonutrients, vitamins, and minerals. This vegetable is a good source of antioxidants, which paired with fiber and different vitamins, makes bok choy an anti-cancer and cholesterol-reducing meal.

Broccoli: Like arugula, broccoli is a cruciferous vegetable and a great source of dietary fiber. It includes vitamin C, which aids aid healing, as well as vitamin E, which may help minimize your risk for some cancers. Broccoli is also rich in iron, potassium, calcium, selenium, zinc, and sulfur.

Brussels Sprout: These veggies are rich in nutritional fiber, folate, potassium, and manganese. A single cup of Brussels sprouts also includes greater than 100 percent of your daily recommended intake of both vitamins C and K. Brussels sprouts have been related to cancer prevention and have also been demonstrated to help detoxification.

Cabbage: Cabbage is one of several foods that naturally contain vitamin E. This vegetable is also high in sulfur, which has been demonstrated to assist cleanse the blood and detoxify the liver. Cabbage also includes bactericidal, antioxidant, and anti-inflammatory effects.

Carrot: Carrots are one of the most commonly accessible veggies, and they are also extraordinarily rich in vitamins and minerals. Carrots are an excellent supply of vitamins A, B, and C as well as iron, calcium, potassium, and sodium. Carrots also include beta-carotene and carotenoids, which aid lower the risk for cancer, cardiovascular disease, and macular degeneration.

Cauliflower: Cauliflower is an extremely versatile vegetable that is also rich in a lot of nutrients. High in B vitamins, phosphorus, potassium, manganese, and vitamin K, this vegetable is particularly nutrition packed. Cauliflower is also a high source of antioxidants as well as glucosinolates, which assist enhance the liver's cleansing abilities.

Celery: A very low-calorie vegetable, celery is rich in a number of vitamins and minerals. The silicon concentration in celery helps to strengthen joints and bones, while iron and magnesium aid promote blood health. Celery has been found to have diuretic and anti-cancer effects.

Cilantro: Cilantro is a plant that is very rich in antioxidants that may help decrease your LDL (bad) cholesterol and boost your good (HDL) cholesterol levels. This plant contains several vitamins, including folate acid, niacin, beta-carotene, and vitamins A, C, and K. There is other data that show that cilantro may be effective in controlling Alzheimer's disease.

Collard Greens: Collard greens are a rich source of vitamin C, manganese, chlorophyll, and beta-carotene. They have both antioxidant and anti-cancer properties. They may also be the strongest of all veggies in decreasing harmful cholesterol levels.

Cucumber: Cucumbers are a rich source of potassium and phytosterols, both of which aid to decrease cholesterol. These veggies have a high water content, which makes them perfect for juicing. They have been a strong source of B vitamins and may help regulate blood pressure.

Dandelion Greens: Though it may seem weird to consume them, dandelion greens are really highly healthful. These greens are a good source of vitamin K, which helps to strengthen blood and bone health. Dandelion greens also include minerals that help to liver and gallbladder health.

Fennel: Fennel is very useful for the digestive system. This plant includes calcium, folate, potassium, magnesium, phosphorus, iron, and copper. It is also a strong source of vitamins C and B5.

Garlic: Garlic is recognized for its antibacterial, antibiotic, and anti-cancer properties. This allium helps to decrease blood cholesterol levels and to control blood sugar. Garlic also contains a number of vitamins, minerals, contains antioxidants, which make it helpful for improving the immune system.

Ginger: Ginger is a good meal for detoxing—it cleanses the body and helps to maintain healthy digestion. Ginger also includes antinausea, anti-inflammatory, and antioxidant properties.

Green Onion: Green onions are sometimes called scallions or spring onions, and they include a number of vitamins and minerals as well as other phytochemicals. These veggies include vitamins K and C, which aid to assist bone health, as well as vitamin A for eye health. Green onions are being a significant source of different phytochemicals like quercetin and anthocyanins, which improve immune system health.

Kale: Kale is the greatest vegetable source of vitamin K, which may aid lessen the risk for some malignancies. This leafy vegetable is also an excellent source of calcium, iron, chlorophyll, and vitamins C and A. Kale is quite nutrition rich, supplying numerous vital minerals, including iron, potassium, phosphorus, and manganese.

Mint: Mint is an herb that helps to alleviate both indigestion and inflammation—its fragrance alone may activate the salivary glands, prompting the synthesis of enzymes that help digestion. Mint is also an excellent source of plant-based omega-3 fatty acids, which maintain healthy hair, skin, and nails.

Parsley: This plant is one of the top natural sources for vitamin C. Parsley is high in folate, which helps to prevent some cancers and may also promote heart health. It also has diuretic characteristics, which implies that it helps the body eliminate extra water.

Parsnip: Parsnips are recognized for its anti-cancer and anti-inflammatory characteristics. These plants provide high quantities of vitamins C and E as well as protein, iron, and calcium. Parsnips have also been utilized as a natural diuretic and detoxifier.

Pumpkin: Pumpkin has been demonstrated to decrease inflammation and may also minimize your risk for prostate cancer. This veggie is strong in vitamins C and E as well as copper, iron, and potassium. The phytochemicals found in pumpkin have also been demonstrated to have a beneficial impact on insulin and glucose levels in diabetic lab models.

Radish: Radishes are the roots of cruciferous vegetables, and they are a good source of vitamins and minerals. The leaves of the plant have more protein, calcium, and vitamin C than the roots, and they have often been used to combat cancer, cure renal issues, and alleviate skin irritation. Radishes are also rich in vitamin C, folic acid, and anthocyanins, which make them useful as a cancer-fighting meal.

Romaine Lettuce: While certain lettuces (like iceberg) are quite low in nutrients, such is not the case with romaine lettuce. This lettuce is very rich in vitamins A, K, and C as well as potassium, iron, magnesium, and manganese.

Spinach: Spinach is a rich source of vitamins A, C, and E, and it also includes significant quantities of calcium, iron, potassium, and protein. Additionally, spinach includes choline, a B-complex nutrient that promotes healthy cognitive function. The iron content in spinach helps to develop healthy blood cells.

Summer Squash: Summer squash is relatively low in calories yet rich in vitamins. These vegetables provide vitamins C and A as well as magnesium, copper, riboflavin, and phosphorus. Summer squash is also an excellent source of antioxidants, which assist to repair damage from free radicals.

Sweet Potato: Sweet potatoes have been found as useful for eye health, detoxification, and digestive assistance. High in copper, iron, magnesium, manganese, and other minerals, sweet potatoes also contain anti-cancer characteristics.

Swiss Chard: A leafy green vegetable, Swiss chard (and other chards), is regarded one of the healthiest veggies available. Chards are rich in dietary fiber and protein in addition to possessing high quantities of vitamins A, K, and C.

Tomato: Tomatoes are a significant source of vitamin C, potassium, copper, iron, and magnesium. They are reported to include over nine thousand phytonutrients, including the antioxidant lycopene, which has been related to cancer prevention and enhanced mental and physical wellness.

Zucchini: Zucchini is an excellent source of copper, iron, magnesium, manganese, phosphorus, potassium, and vitamin C. This veggie is also a rich source of vitamin A and niacin (vitamin B3), which has been related to lower risk for cardiovascular disease.

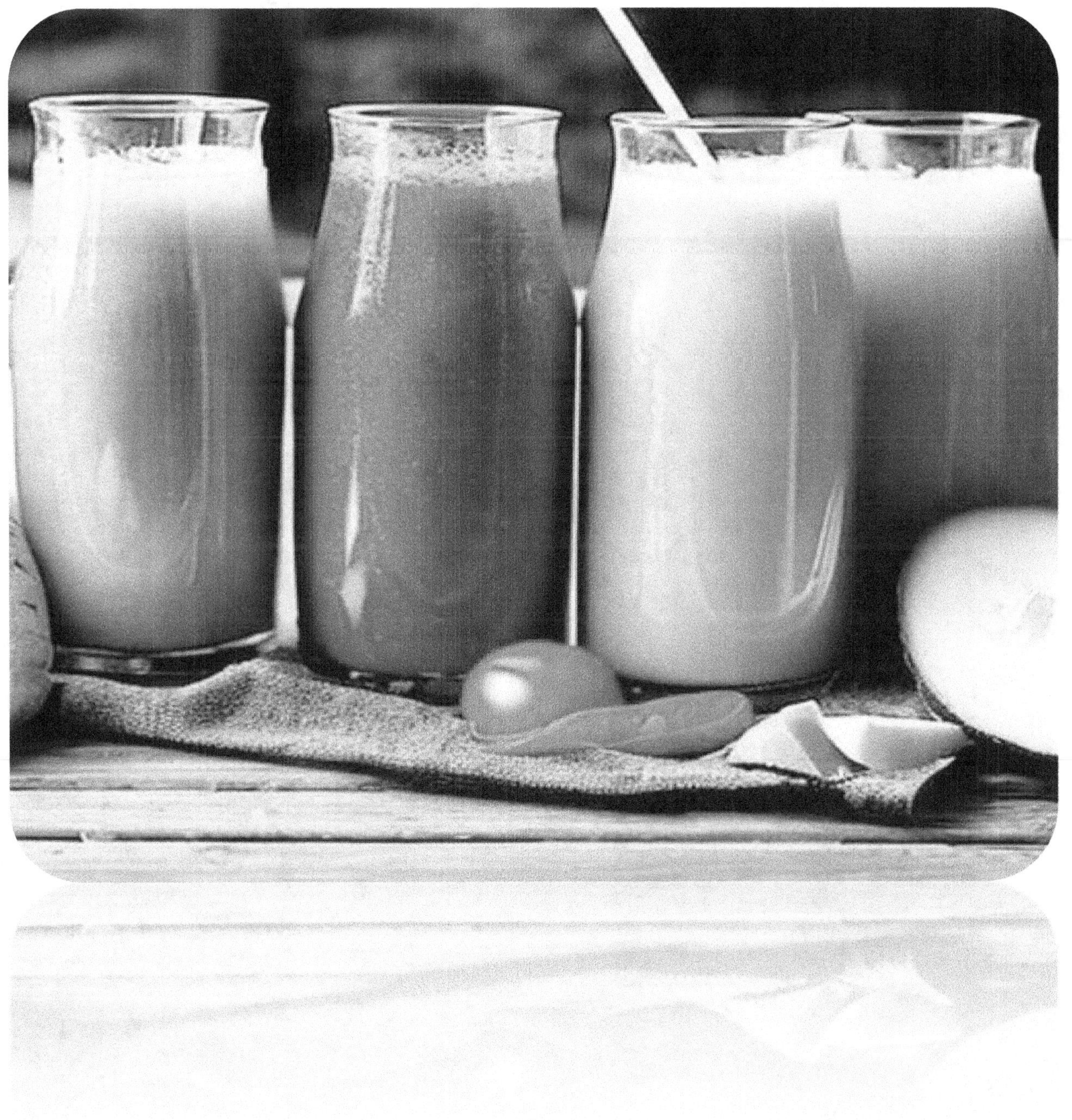

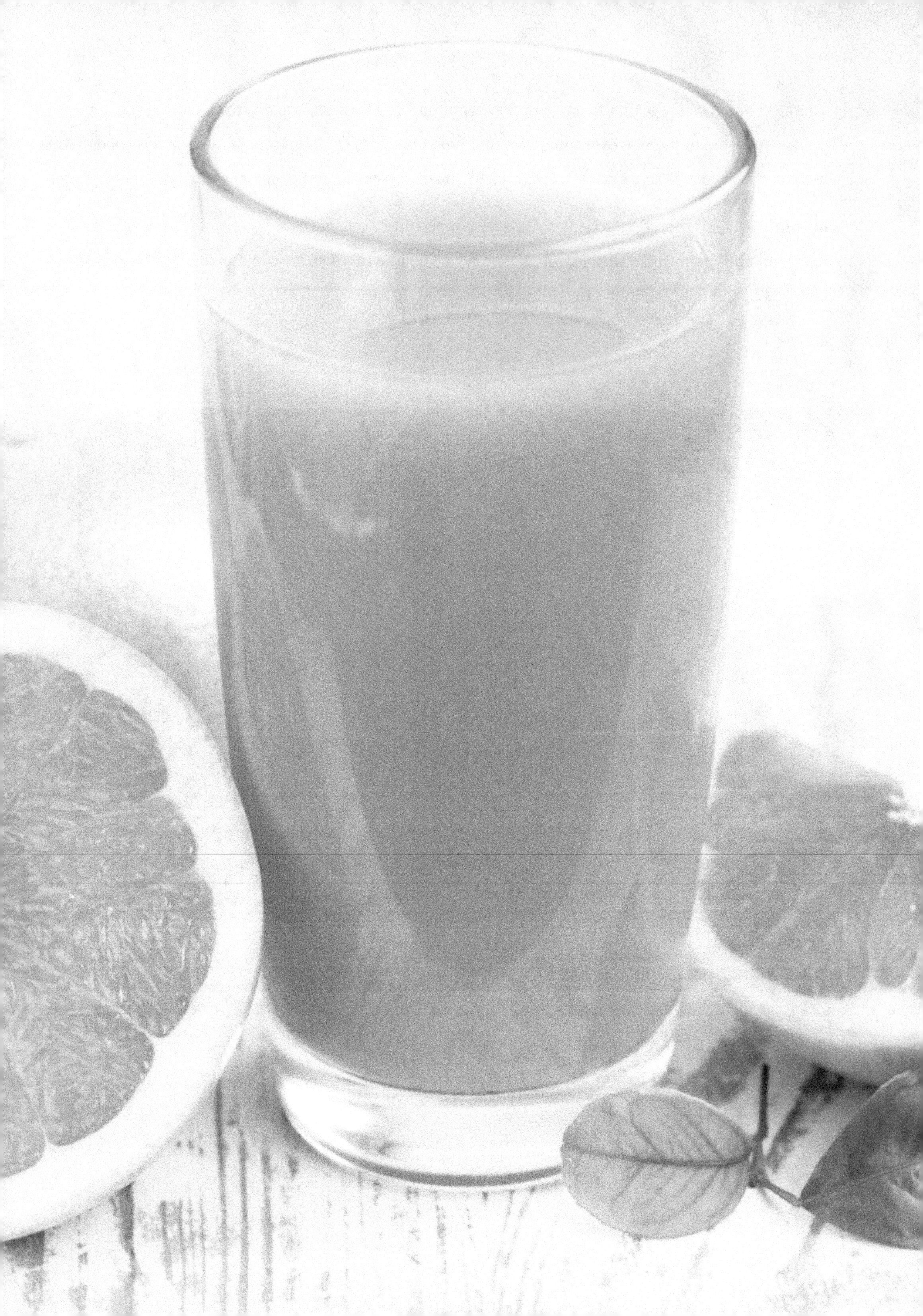

7-DAYS MEAL PLAN

Day	Breakfast	Lunch	Dinner	Substitutions
1	Dreamy Green Juice	Jolly Green Giant Juice with grilled chicken salad (spinach, romaine, carrots, chickpeas, vinaigrette)	Beets Me Blend with baked salmon and roasted Brussels sprouts	Green juice: Sensibly Sweet Juice; Salad protein: tofu, tuna; Dinner: Seven-Layer Green Juice, chicken breast
2	Refreshing Green Juice	Double Trouble Broccoli Juice with turkey and vegetable wrap (whole-wheat tortilla, lettuce, tomato, cucumber, hummus)	Beautiful Beet Juice with lentil soup and whole-wheat bread	Green juice: Lean, Mean Green Juice; Wrap fillings: black beans, avocado; Dinner: Roasted chicken, quinoa
3	Easy Peasy Green Lemonade (if details provided)	Green Goodness Juice with quinoa bowl (quinoa, black beans, roasted peppers, corn, salsa)	Deeply Green Juice with shrimp scampi and brown rice	Green lemonade: Simply Sweet Green Juice; Bowl toppings: avocado, cheese, sour cream; Dinner: Grilled salmon, roasted vegetables
4	Mango Tango Green Juice	Tossed Salad Juice with whole-wheat crackers and hummus	Seven-Layer Green Juice with lentil soup and whole-wheat bread	Green juice: Jolly Green Giant Juice; Salad: add chicken/tuna; Dinner: Baked tofu, stir-fried vegetables
5	Rocket Fuel Green Juice	Spicy Green Juice with black bean burger on whole-wheat bun and side salad	Beets Me Blend with roasted chicken breast and sweet potato	Green juice: Deeply Green Juice; Burger toppings: avocado, cheese, lettuce; Dinner: Baked salmon, quinoa
6	Sensibly Sweet Juice	Lean, Mean Green Juice with tuna salad sandwich on whole-wheat bread	Double Trouble Broccoli Juice with brown rice and stir-fried tofu and vegetables	Green juice: Refreshing Green Juice; Sandwich fillings: chicken salad, egg salad; Dinner: Grilled chicken, roasted Brussels sprouts
7	Jolly Green Giant Juice	Beautiful Beet Juice with grilled fish and steamed vegetables	Seven-Layer Green Juice with lentil soup and whole-wheat bread	Green juice: Mango Tango Green Juice; Fish: salmon, cod; Vegetables: broccoli, asparagus; Dinner: Grilled chicken breast, roasted sweet potato

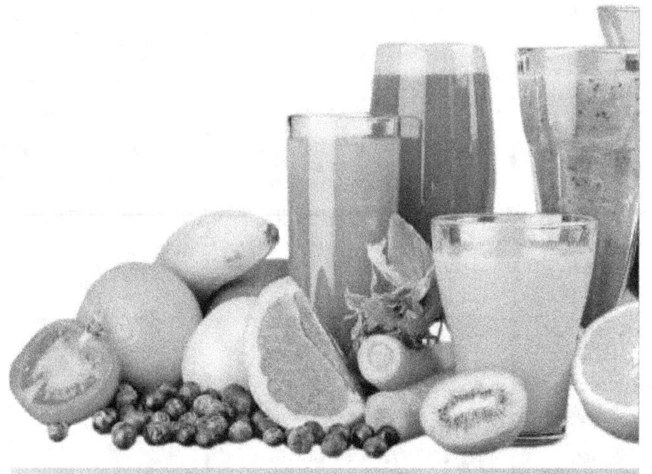

ADDITIONAL TIPS

Breakfast: Substitute green juices with smoothies, fruit with yogurt, or whole-wheat toast with avocado.

Lunch: Consider protein options like grilled chicken, fish, tofu, or beans. Add whole-wheat crackers, fruit, or yogurt for variety.

Dinner: Explore different lean protein sources like chicken, fish, tofu, or lentils. Substitute roasted vegetables with steamed or stir-fried options.

Snacks: Include fruits, vegetables, nuts, yogurt, or whole-wheat crackers throughout the day.

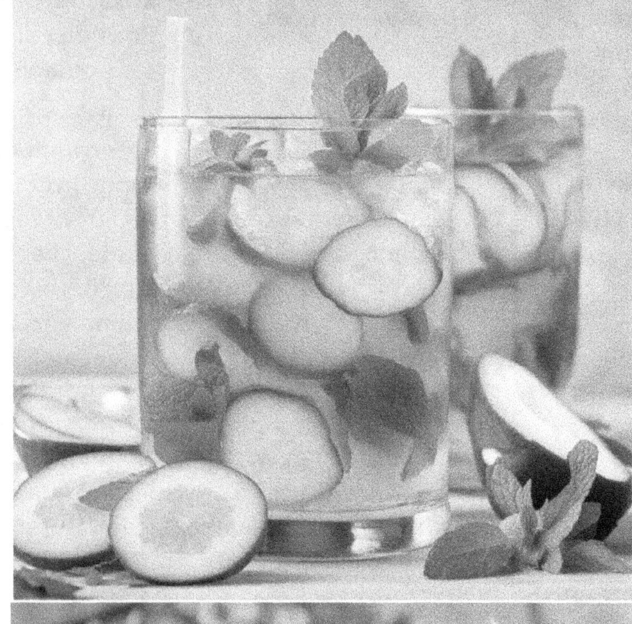

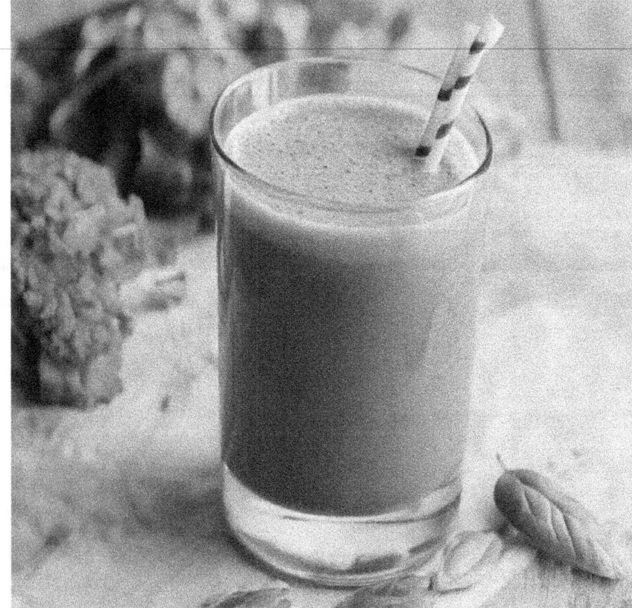

FRUIT JUICE

While often enjoyed for their refreshing taste and vibrant colors, fruit juice recipes offer more than just a burst of sweetness. They can be a convenient way to pack your diet with essential nutrients:

Vitamins and minerals: Fruits are powerhouses of vitamins like C, A, and K, along with minerals like potassium and magnesium, all crucial for various bodily functions.

Antioxidants: Many fruits are loaded with antioxidant compounds that help fight free radicals and protect your cells from damage.

Dietary fiber: Some fruits, like berries, provide fiber, which aids in digestion and gut health.

Hydration: Juices contribute to your daily fluid intake, especially when combined with water.

However, it's important to remember:

Sugar content: Fruits are naturally sweet, and juices concentrate that sweetness. Moderation is key to avoid excessive sugar intake.

Fiber loss: Juicing removes most of the fiber from fruits, which can impact digestion and nutrient absorption.

Not a substitute for whole fruits: Juices lack the whole fruit's texture, fiber, and satiety benefits. Enjoy them as a supplement, not a replacement.

By incorporating a variety of fruits and mindful consumption, fruit juice recipes can be a delicious and nutritious addition to your diet!

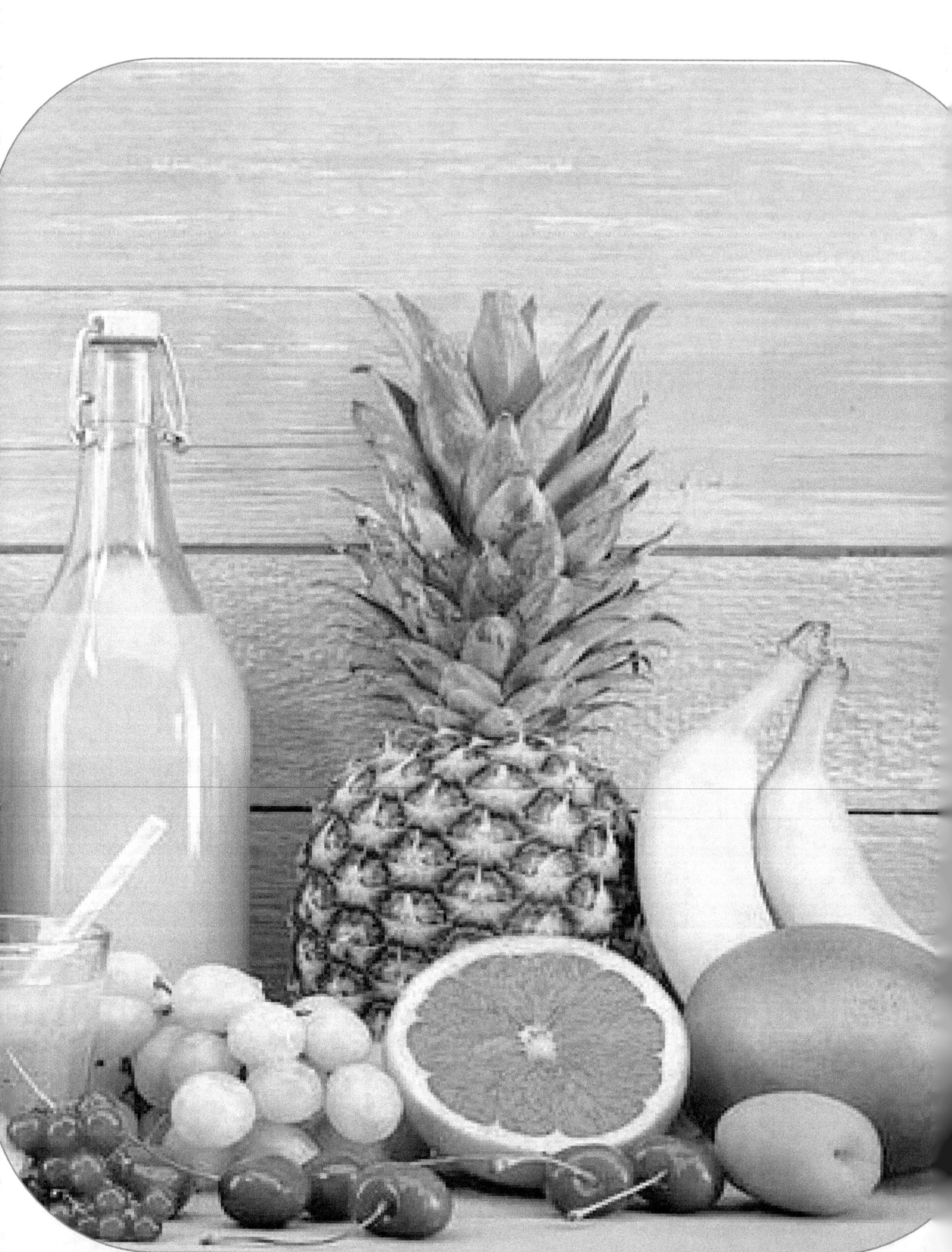

FRUIT JUICE RECIPES:

Energy Explosion Juice

Prep Time: 5 minutes

Servings: 1

NUTRITIONAL VALUES:

- Calories: 140
- Carbs: 30g
- Sugar: 25g
- Fiber: 3g
- Vitamin C: 140% DV

INGREDIENTS:

- 1 apple, cored and cut
- 1 grapefruit, peeled and sliced
- 1 lemon, peeled and quartered
- 1-inch ginger root, peeled and sliced (optional)
- 1/2 cup spinach leaves

INSTRUCTIONS:

1. Wash and prepare all fruits and ginger.
2. Feed materials into your juicer in the following order: apple, grapefruit, lemon, ginger (if using), spinach.
3. Stir or shake the juice thoroughly and drink immediately.

Tips:

1. This juice is naturally sweet and tangy.

2. Adjust the lemon or grapefruit quantity to your taste choice.
3. For an added zing, add a sprinkle of cayenne pepper.

Sparkling Kiwi Pineapple Juice

Prep Time: 5 minutes

Servings: 1

NUTRITIONAL VALUES:

- Calories: 130
- Carbs: 32g
- Sugar: 30g
- Fiber: 2g
- Vitamin C: 220% DV

INGREDIENTS:

- 2 kiwis, peeled and chopped
- 1/2 pineapple, cored and chopped
- 1/2 lime, juiced
- 1/4 cup sparkling water

INSTRUCTIONS:

1. Wash and prepare kiwi and pineapple.
2. Juice the kiwi and pineapple together.
3. Add lime juice and mix thoroughly.
4. Pour into a glass and top with sparkling water.
5. Serve immediately.

1. You may add fresh lime wedges for garnish and an extra punch of citrus flavor.

Mango Melon Juice

Prep Time: 5 minutes

Servings: 1

NUTRITIONAL VALUES:

- Calories: 120
- Carbs: 28g
- Sugar: 25g
- Fiber: 2g
- Vitamin A: 130% DV

INGREDIENTS:

- 1/2 mango, pitted and chopped
- 1 cup cantaloupe, cubed
- 1/2 cup honeydew melon, cubed
- 1/4 cup fresh mint leaves

INSTRUCTIONS:

2. Wash and prepare mango and melons.
3. Juice the mango and cantaloupe together.
4. Add honeydew melon and mint leaves to the juicer and process again.
5. Stir thoroughly and enjoy immediately.

Tip:

1. For a thicker consistency, remove part of the melody liquid before adding the mint leaves.

Strawberry Lemonade Juice

Prep Time: 5 minutes

Servings: 1

NUTRITIONAL VALUES:

- Calories: 110
- Carbs: 25g
- Sugar: 20g
- Vitamin C: 130% DV

INGREDIENTS:

- 1 cup strawberries, hulled
- 1/2 lemon, juiced
- 1/4 cup water
- 1 tablespoon honey (optional)

INSTRUCTIONS:

1. Wash and hull strawberries.
2. Juice the strawberries with lemon juice.
3. Add water and honey (if using) and whisk thoroughly.
4. Pour into a glass and drink immediately.

Tip:

1. Use frozen strawberries for a richer and cooler juice.

2. For a bubbly variation, top with some club soda.

Berry Mint Blast

Prep Time: 5 minutes

Servings: 1

NUTRITIONAL VALUES:

- Calories: 80
- Carbs: 18g
- Sugar: 15g
- Fiber: 3g
- Vitamin C: 150% DV

INGREDIENTS:

- 1 cup mixed berries (blueberries, raspberries, strawberries)
- 1/2 cucumber, peeled and cut
- 1/4 cup fresh mint leaves
- 1/4 cup water

INSTRUCTIONS:

1. Wash and prepare all ingredients.
2. Juice the berries and cucumber together.
3. Add mint leaves and water to the juicer and process again.
4. Stir thoroughly and enjoy immediately.

Tip:

1. For a more powerful mint taste, you may muddle the mint leaves in the bottom of the glass before adding the juice.

Morning Melon Boost

Prep Time: 5 minutes

Servings: 1

NUTRITIONAL VALUES:

- Calories: 100
- Carbs: 22g
- Sugar: 20g
- Fiber: 2g
- Vitamin C: 120% DV

INGREDIENTS:

- 1/2 cantaloupe, cubed
- 1/2 honeydew melon, cubed
- 1/4 cup pineapple, diced
- 1/2 lime, juiced
- 1-inch ginger root, peeled and minced (optional)

INSTRUCTIONS:

2. Wash and prepare all fruits and ginger.
3. Juice the cantaloupe, honeydew melon, and pineapple together.
4. Add lime juice and ginger (if using) and whisk thoroughly.
5. Serve immediately.

Tip:

1. This drink is naturally sweet and refreshing.
2. For an added kick, add a sprinkle of cayenne pepper or a few basil leaves.

Tutti-Frutti Juice

Prep Time: 5 minutes

Servings: 1

NUTRITIONAL VALUES:

- Calories: 150
- Carbs: 35g
- Sugar: 30g
- Fiber: 3g
- Vitamin C: 180% DV

INGREDIENTS:

- 1/2 cup mixed berries (blueberries, raspberries, strawberries)
- 1/2 mango, pitted and cut
- 1/4 cup pineapple, chopped
- 1/4 cup orange, peeled and segmented
- 1/2 lime, juiced

INSTRUCTIONS:

1. Wash and prepare all fruits.
2. Juice the berries, mango, and pineapple together.
3. Add orange segments and lime juice to the juicer and process again.
4. Stir thoroughly and enjoy immediately.

Tip:

1. This juice is rich with taste and minerals.
2. You may alter the fruit mix according on your desire.

Easy Apple Celery Juice

Prep Time: 5 minutes

Servings: 1

NUTRITIONAL VALUES:

- Calories: 80
- Carbs: 18g
- Sugar: 15g
- Fiber: 3g
- Vitamin C: 20% DV

INGREDIENTS:

- 1 apple, cored and chopped
- 2 celery stalks, chopped
- 1/2 lemon, juiced

INSTRUCTIONS:

1. Wash and prepare apple and celery.
2. Juice the apple and celery together.
3. Add lemon juice and mix thoroughly.
4. Serve immediately.

Tip:

1. This simple drink is a terrific way to get your daily dosage of vitamins and fiber.

2. For a sweeter taste, add a few slices of pear or grapes.

Blueberry Beet Juice

Prep Time: 5 minutes

Servings: 1

NUTRITIONAL VALUES:

- Calories: 90
- Carbs: 20g
- Sugar: 18g
- Fiber: 3g
- Vitamin C: 25% DV

INGREDIENTS:

- 1 cup blueberries
- 1/2 beet, peeled and chopped
- 1/2 apple, cored and chopped
- 1/2 lemon, juiced

INSTRUCTIONS:

1. Wash and prepare all ingredients.
2. Juice the blueberries and beet together.
3. Add apple and lemon juice to the juicer and process again.
4. Stir thoroughly and enjoy immediately.

Tip:

1. This earthy and vibrant juice is rich in antioxidants and nutrients.

2. If you find the best flavor too strong, add more apple or another mild-flavored fruit.

Tropical Dream Juice

Prep Time: 5 minutes

Servings: 1

NUTRITIONAL VALUES:

- Calories: 140
- Carbs: 32g
- Sugar: 30g
- Fiber: 2g
- Vitamin C: 150% DV

INGREDIENTS:

- 1/2 pineapple, cored and chopped
- 1/2 papaya, peeled and seeded
- 1/4 cup orange, peeled and segmented
- 1/4 cup mango, pitted and chopped
- 1/2 lime, juiced

INSTRUCTIONS:

1. Wash and prepare all ingredients.
2. Juice the pineapple, papaya, and orange together.
3. Add mango and lime juice to the juicer and process again.
4. Stir thoroughly and enjoy immediately.

Tip:

1. For a creamier texture, add a dollop of plain yogurt or coconut milk before blending.

Green Glow Up Juice

Prep Time: 5 minutes

Servings: 1

NUTRITIONAL VALUES:

- Calories: 80
- Carbs: 15g
- Sugar: 10g
- Fiber: 4g
- Vitamin C: 120% DV

INGREDIENTS:

- 1 cucumber, peeled and chopped
- 1 apple, cored and cut
- 1 handful spinach leaves
- 1 handful kale leaves
- 1/2 lemon, juiced

INSTRUCTIONS:

2. Wash and prepare all ingredients.
3. Juice the cucumber and apple together.
4. Add spinach, kale, and lemon juice to the juicer and process again.
5. Stir thoroughly and enjoy immediately.

Tip:

1. This juice is a great way to get your daily dose of greens and essential vitamins.
2. For a sweeter taste, add a few slices of pear or grapes.

Citrus Sunshine Juice

Prep Time: 5 minutes

Servings: 1

NUTRITIONAL VALUES:

- Calories: 70
- Carbs: 15g
- Sugar: 12g
- Fiber: 2g
- Vitamin C: 200% DV

INGREDIENTS:

- 1 grapefruit, peeled and sliced
- 1 orange, peeled and segmented
- 1/2 lemon, juiced
- 1/2-inch ginger root, peeled and chopped (optional)

INSTRUCTIONS:

1. Wash and prepare all ingredients.
2. Juice the grapefruit and orange together.
3. Add lemon juice and ginger (if using) and stir well.
4. Serve immediately.

Tip:

1. This invigorating juice is packed with vitamin C and antioxidants.

2. It's a perfect way to start your day or boost your energy throughout the day.

Berrylicious Blast Juice

Prep Time: 5 minutes

Servings: 1

NUTRITIONAL VALUES:

- Calories: 120
- Carbs: 28g
- Sugar: 25g
- Fiber: 3g
- Vitamin C: 130% DV

INGREDIENTS:

- 1 cup mixed berries (blueberries, raspberries, strawberries)
- 1/2 banana, peeled and frozen
- 1/4 cup Greek yogurt
- 1/4 cup almond milk
- 1/2 teaspoon honey (optional)

INSTRUCTIONS:

1. Wash and prepare berries.
2. Blend all ingredients together in a blender until smooth.
3. Pour into a glass and drink immediately.

Tip:

1. This smoothie-like juice is a delicious and nutritious way to incorporate protein and healthy fats into your diet.

2. The frozen banana adds thickness and creaminess.

Watermelon Cooler Juice

Prep Time: 5 minutes

Servings: 1

NUTRITIONAL VALUES:

- Calories: 70
- Carbs: 16g
- Sugar: 15g
- Fiber: 1g
- Vitamin C: 25% DV

INGREDIENTS:

- 2 cups seedless watermelon, cubed
- 1/2 cucumber, peeled and chopped
- 1/4 cup mint leaves
- 1/4 lime, juiced

INSTRUCTIONS:

1. Wash and prepare all ingredients.
2. Juice the watermelon and cucumber together.
3. Add mint leaves and lime juice to the juicer and process again.
4. Pour into a glass with ice and enjoy immediately.

Cilantro Strawberry Banana Juice

Prep Time: 5 minutes

Servings: 1

NUTRITIONAL VALUES:

- Calories: 180
- Carbs: 40g
- Sugar: 35g
- Fiber: 3g
- Vitamin C: 100% DV

INGREDIENTS:

- 1 cup strawberries, hulled
- 1/2 banana, peeled
- 1/4 cup fresh cilantro leaves
- 1/4 cup water
- 1/2 lime, juiced (optional)

INSTRUCTIONS:

1. Wash and prepare all ingredients.
2. Juice the strawberries and banana together.
3. Add cilantro leaves, water, and lime juice (if using) to the juicer and process again.
4. Stir thoroughly and enjoy immediately.

Blackberry Kiwi Juice Blend

Prep Time: 5 minutes

Servings: 1

NUTRITIONAL VALUES:

- Calories: 120
- Carbs: 28g
- Sugar: 25g
- Fiber: 3g
- Vitamin C: 220% DV

INGREDIENTS:

- 1 cup blackberries
- 1 kiwi, peeled and cut
- 1/2 apple, cored and cut
- 1/4 cup water
- 1/2 teaspoon honey (optional)

INSTRUCTIONS:

1. Wash and prepare all ingredients.

2. Blend all ingredients together in a blender until smooth.

3. Pour into a glass and drink immediately.

<u>Tip:</u>

1. This creamy and tangy combination is filled with vitamin C and antioxidants.

2. Feel free to modify the sweetness with honey or another natural sweetener.

Orange-Carrot Ginger Juice

Prep Time: 5 minutes

Servings: 1

NUTRITIONAL VALUES:

- Calories: 100
- Carbs: 22g
- Sugar: 20g
- Fiber: 3g
- Vitamin A: 230% DV

INGREDIENTS:

- 1 orange, peeled and segmented
- 1 carrot, peeled and sliced
- 1/2-inch ginger root, peeled and sliced
- 1/2 lemon, juiced

INSTRUCTIONS:

1. Wash and prepare all ingredients.

2. Juice the orange and carrot together.

3. Add ginger and lemon juice to the juicer and process again.

4. Stir thoroughly and enjoy immediately.

<u>Tip:</u>

1. This revitalizing drink is rich in vitamins and minerals, encouraging good immune function and eyesight.

2. For a milder ginger taste, use a smaller slice.

Sparkling Raspberry Pomegranate Juice

Prep Time: 5 minutes

Servings: 1

NUTRITIONAL VALUES:

- Calories: 130
- Carbs: 30g
- Sugar: 25g
- Fiber: 3g
- Vitamin C: 80% DV

INGREDIENTS:

- 1 cup raspberries
- 1/2 pomegranate, seeds removed
- 1/4 cup apple, cored and chopped (optional)
- 1/4 cup sparkling water
- 1/4 lime, juiced (optional)

1. Wash and prepare all ingredients.
2. Juice the raspberries and apple (if using) together.
3. Add pomegranate seeds and lime juice (if used) to the juicer and process again.
4. Pour into a glass and top with sparkling water.
5. Serve immediately.

Tip:

1. This colorful juice is naturally sweet and effervescent, great for a refreshing pick-me-up.
2. Adjust the fruit mix for varied taste variations.

Pineapple Lavender Juice

Prep Time: 5 minutes

Servings: 1

NUTRITIONAL VALUES:

- Calories: 120
- Carbs: 28g
- Sugar: 25g
- Fiber: 2g
- Vitamin C: 130% DV

INGREDIENTS:

- 1/2 pineapple, cored and cut
- 1 bunch fresh lavender sprigs
- 1/2 cucumber, peeled and cut
- 1/4 lime, juiced
- 1/4 cup water (optional)

INSTRUCTIONS:

1. Wash and prepare all ingredients.
2. Muddle the lavender sprigs in the bottom of a glass.
3. Juice the pineapple and cucumber together.
4. Add lime juice and water (if using) to the juicer and process again.
5. Strain the juice and pour it into the glass with the muddled lavender.
6. Enjoy instantly.

Tip:

1. Lavender provides a gentle flowery scent to this drink.
2. Don't over-muddle since it might turn bitter.
3. For a greater lavender taste, you may infuse the water with dried lavender beforehand.

Pretty in Pink Juice Blend

Prep Time: 5 minutes

Servings: 1

NUTRITIONAL VALUES:

- Calories: 130

- Carbs: 30g
- Sugar: 25g
- Fiber: 3g
- Vitamin C: 140% DV

INGREDIENTS:

- 1 cup raspberries
- 1/2 grapefruit, peeled and sliced
- 1/4 cup strawberry, hulled
- 1/4 cup watermelon, diced
- 1/4 cup coconut water

INSTRUCTIONS:

1. Wash and prepare all ingredients.
2. Blend all ingredients together in a blender until smooth.
3. Pour into a glass and drink immediately.

Tip:

1. This bright combination is naturally sweet and rich with antioxidants. It's a gorgeous and refreshing treat!

Fruity Green Juice

Prep Time: 5 minutes

Servings: 1

NUTRITIONAL VALUES:

- Calories: 80
- Carbs: 18g
- Sugar: 15g

- Fiber: 4g
- Vitamin C: 120% DV

INGREDIENTS:

- 1 cucumber, peeled and cut
- 1 apple, cored and cut
- 1 bunch spinach leaves
- 1 handful kale leaves
- 1/2 lemon, juiced
- 1/4 cup pineapple, chopped (optional)

INSTRUCTIONS:

2. Wash and prepare all ingredients.
3. Juice the cucumber and apple together.
4. Add spinach, kale, lemon juice, and pineapple (if using) to the juicer and process again.
5. Stir thoroughly and enjoy immediately.

Tip:

1. This green juice is a terrific way to get your daily dosage of greens and critical vitamins.
2. The pineapple provides a bit of sweetness if desired.

Papaya Pineapple Juice Blend

Prep Time: 5 minutes

Servings: 1

NUTRITIONAL VALUES:

- Calories: 150
- Carbs: 35g
- Sugar: 30g
- Fiber: 2g
- Vitamin C: 200% DV

INGREDIENTS:

- 1/2 papaya, peeled and seeded
- 1/2 pineapple, cored and cut
- 1/4 lime, juiced
- 1/4 cup unsweetened coconut milk (optional)

INSTRUCTIONS:

1. Wash and prepare all ingredients.
2. Blend the papaya and pineapple together until smooth.
3. Add lime juice and coconut milk (if using) and mix again until thoroughly integrated.
4. Pour into a glass and drink immediately.

Tip:

1. This creamy and tropical combination is packed in vitamins and antioxidants.
2. The coconut milk gives a wonderful touch of creaminess and healthful fats.

Cucumber Melon Juice

Prep Time: 5 minutes

Servings: 1

NUTRITIONAL VALUES:

- Calories: 70
- Carbs: 14g
- Sugar: 12g
- Fiber: 1g
- Vitamin C: 20% DV

INGREDIENTS:

- 1 cucumber, peeled and cut
- 1 cup cantaloupe, cubed
- 1/2 honeydew melon, diced
- 1/4 cup mint leaves
- 1/4 lime, juiced

INSTRUCTIONS:

1. Wash and prepare all ingredients.
2. Juice the cucumber and melons together.
3. Add mint leaves and lime juice to the juicer and process again.
4. Stir thoroughly and enjoy immediately.

Tip:

1. This cool beverage is excellent for a hot summer day.
2. The mint lends a lovely freshness while the melons produce a naturally sweet taste.

Blueberry Beauty Juice

Prep Time: 5 minutes

Servings: 1

- Calories: 110
- Carbs: 25g
- Sugar: 20g
- Fiber: 3g
- Vitamin C: 130% DV

INGREDIENTS:

- 1 cup blueberries
- 1/2 apple, cored and cut
- 1/2 banana, peeled
- 1/4 cup Greek yogurt
- 1/4 cup almond milk
- 1/2 teaspoon chia seeds

INSTRUCTIONS:

1. Wash and prepare all ingredients.
2. Blend all ingredients together in a blender until smooth.
3. Pour into a glass and top with chia seeds.

Tip:

1. This protein-rich and creamy combination is filled with antioxidants and healthy fats.
2. It's a tasty and healthy way to start your day or replenish after a workout.

Razzle Dazzle Berry Juice

Prep Time: 5 minutes

Servings: 1

NUTRITIONAL VALUES:

- Calories: 140
- Carbs: 32g
- Sugar: 30g
- Fiber: 3g
- Vitamin C: 180% DV

INGREDIENTS:

- 1/2 cup raspberries
- 1/2 cup blueberries
- 1/4 cup strawberries, hulled
- 1/4 cup blackberries
- 1/2 apple, cored and cut
- 1/4 cup water (optional)

INSTRUCTIONS:

1. Wash and prepare all ingredients.
2. Juice the apple and berries together.
3. Add water (if using) and whisk thoroughly.
4. Pour into a glass and drink immediately.

Tip:

1. This colorful juice explodes with taste and antioxidants from a variety of berries.
2. Adjust the water content to your desired consistency.

Tropical Fruit Juice Blend

Prep Time: 5 minutes

Servings: 1

<u>NUTRITIONAL VALUES:</u>

- Calories: 160
- Carbs: 38g
- Sugar: 35g
- Fiber: 2g
- Vitamin C: 150% DV

<u>INGREDIENTS:</u>

- 1/2 mango, pitted and cut
- 1/2 pineapple, cored and cut
- 1/4 papaya, peeled and seeded
- 1/4 orange, peeled and sliced
- 1/4 lime, juiced

<u>INSTRUCTIONS:</u>

1. Wash and prepare all ingredients.
2. Blend all ingredients together in a blender until smooth.
3. Pour into a glass and drink immediately.

Tip:

1. This creamy and tropical combination is a taste of paradise! The mix of sweet and tart fruits is tempting.

Melon Agua Fresca

Prep Time: 5 minutes

Servings: 1

<u>NUTRITIONAL VALUES:</u>

- Calories: 70
- Carbs: 16g
- Sugar: 15g
- Fiber: 1g
- Vitamin C: 25% DV

<u>INGREDIENTS:</u>

- 2 cups seedless watermelon, cubed
- 1/2 cucumber, peeled and cut
- 1/4 cup fresh mint leaves
- 1/4 lime, juiced
- Pinch of sea salt (optional)

<u>INSTRUCTIONS:</u>

2. Wash and prepare all ingredients.
3. Puree the watermelon and cucumber in a blender until smooth.
4. Strain the mixture through a fine-mesh sieve to remove any pulp.
5. Stir in mint leaves, lime juice, and sea salt (if using).
6. Pour into a glass with ice and drink immediately.

Tip:

1. This refreshing and hydrating drink is excellent for a hot summer day.
2. The mint gives a beautiful scent and the sea salt accentuates the natural sweetness of the melons.

Purple Peach Parsley Juice

Prep Time: 5 minutes

Servings: 1

NUTRITIONAL VALUES:

- Calories: 80
- Carbs: 18g
- Sugar: 15g
- Fiber: 2g
- Vitamin C: 20% DV

INGREDIENTS:

- 1 peach, pitted and chopped
- 1/2 cup blueberries
- 1 bunch fresh parsley leaves
- 1/2 lemon, juiced
- 1/4 cup water (optional)

INSTRUCTIONS:

1. Wash and prepare all ingredients.
2. Juice the peach and blueberries together.
3. Add parsley leaves and lemon juice to the juicer and process again.
4. Add water (if using) and whisk thoroughly.
5. Pour into a glass and drink immediately.

Tip:

1. This unusual juice mix gives a balance of sweet, tart, and earthy tastes.
2. The parsley offers an unexpected flavor and enhances the nutritious value.

Jicama Pear Juice

Prep Time: 5 minutes

Servings: 1

NUTRITIONAL VALUES:

- Calories: 80
- Carbs: 18g
- Sugar: 15g
- Fiber: 3g
- Vitamin C: 30% DV

INGREDIENTS:

- 1 jicama, peeled and chopped
- 1 pear, cored and cut
- 1/2 cucumber, peeled and cut
- 1/4 lime, juiced
- 1/4 cup water (optional)

INSTRUCTIONS:

1. Wash and prepare all ingredients.
2. Juice the jicama, pear, and cucumber together.
3. Add lime juice and water (if using) to the juicer and process again.
4. Stir thoroughly and enjoy immediately.

Tip:

1. This delightful drink is light and low in calories.

2. The jicama lends a distinct, somewhat sweet and crunchy taste, while the pear delivers natural sweetness.

3. The cucumber cools down the flavor and gives hydration.

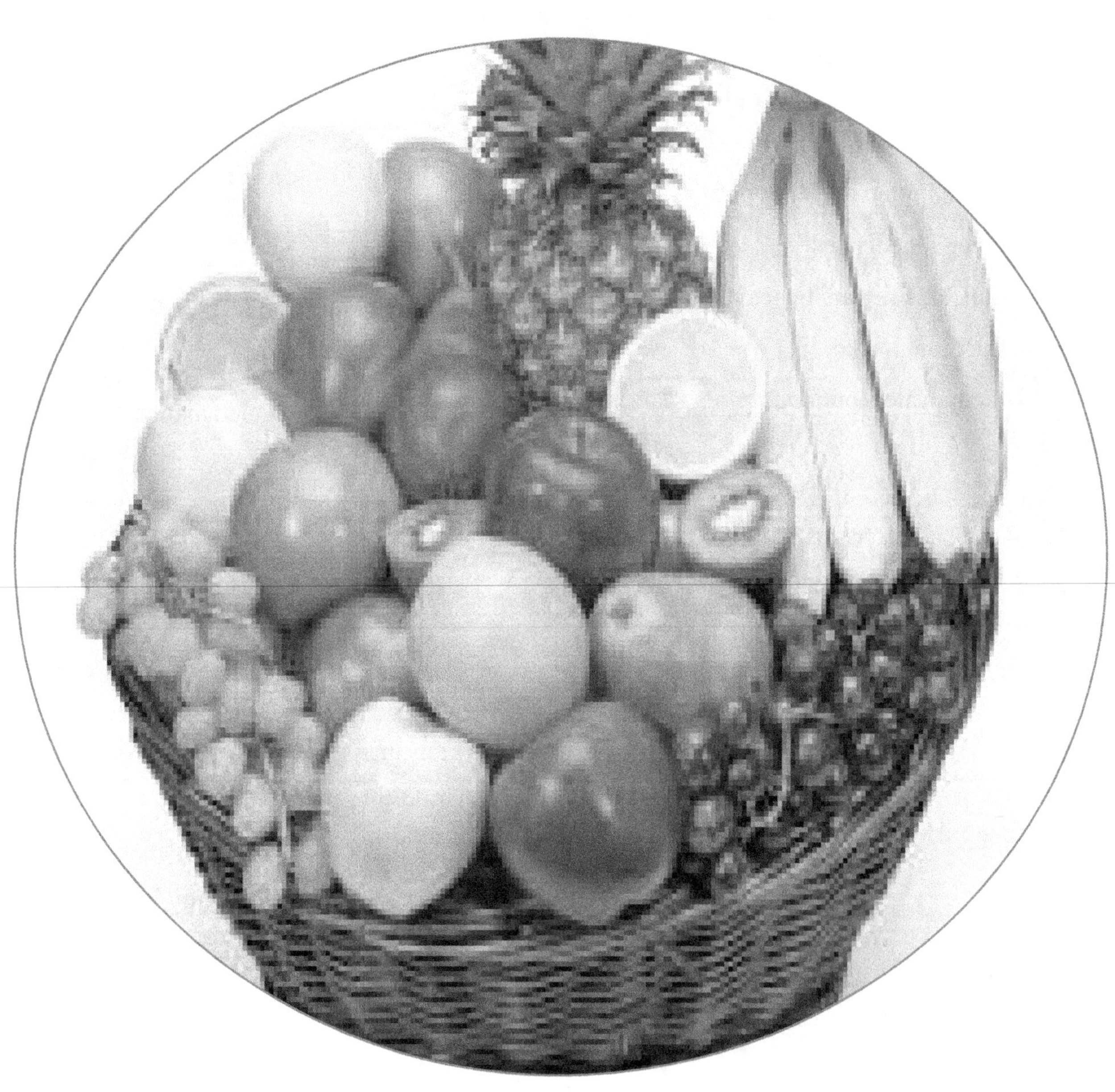

VEGETABLE JUICE

Don't underestimate the humble vegetable juice! Beyond their vibrant hues and earthy appeal, these recipes unlock a treasure trove of nutritional benefits:

Vitamin and mineral bonanza: From vitamin C boosting immunity to potassium regulating blood pressure, vegetable juices offer a spectrum of essential nutrients.

Antioxidant powerhouse: Loaded with plant compounds, they help combat free radicals and contribute to cellular health.

Digestive delight: Many greens and vegetables are rich in fiber, aiding digestion and gut health.

Hydration hero: Juices contribute to your daily fluid intake, keeping you refreshed and energized.

However, remember:

Sugar content: Some blends might contain naturally occurring sugars, so mindful consumption is key.

Limited protein and fat: They focus on vitamins and minerals, so pair them with protein and healthy fats for a balanced meal.

Not a complete meal: Enjoy them alongside other foods for a well-rounded diet.

By choosing diverse vegetables and practicing moderation, vegetable juice recipes can be a powerful tool for enhancing your well-being. So, go green and unlock the goodness!

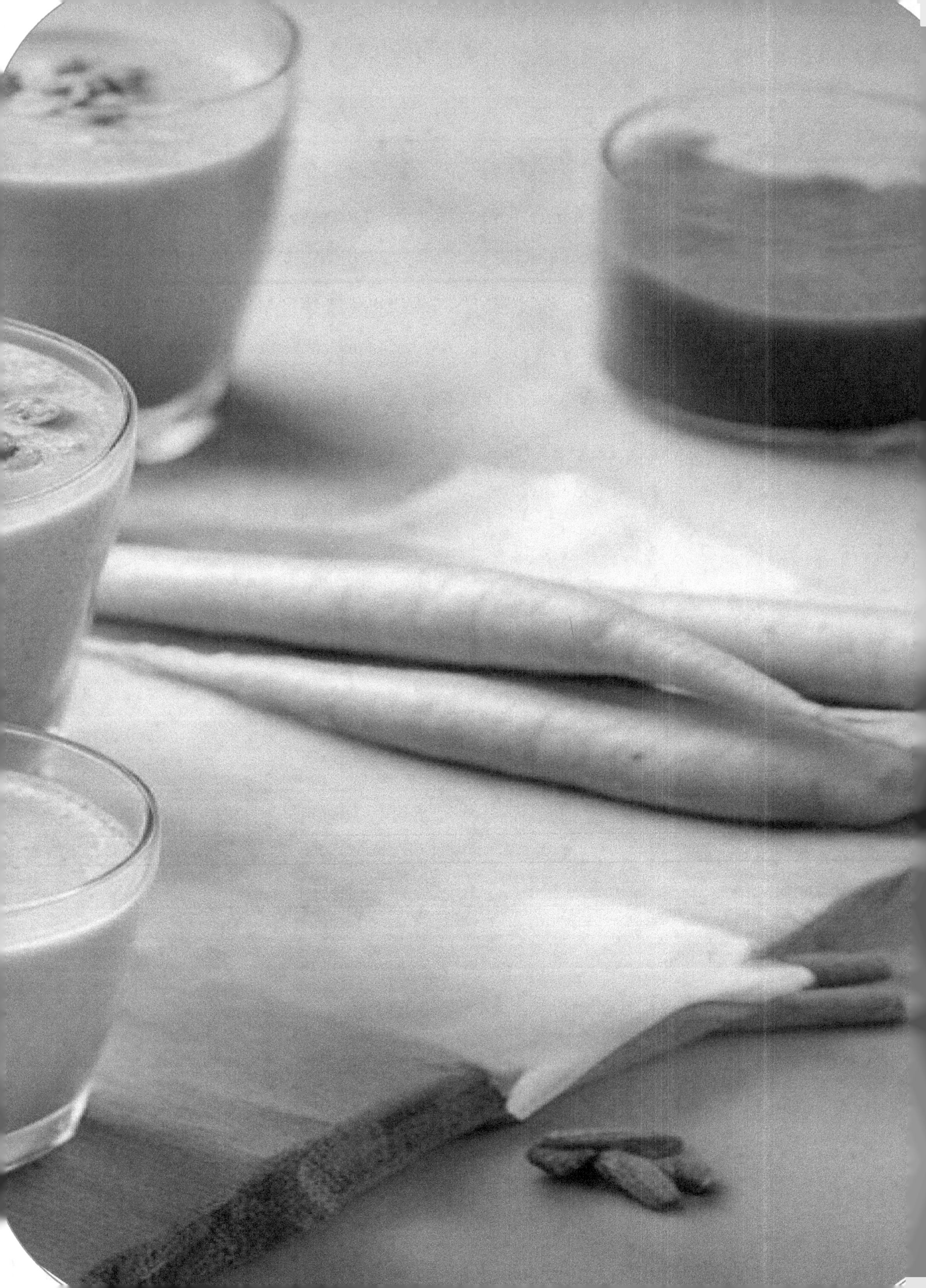

VEGETABLE JUICE RECIPES:

Tomato Gazpacho Juice

Prep Time: 5 minutes

Servings: 1

<u>NUTRITIONAL VALUES:</u>

- Calories: 80
- Carbs: 14g
- Sugar: 10g
- Fiber: 2g
- Vitamin C: 60% DV

<u>INGREDIENTS:</u>

- 1 big tomato, cored and cut
- 1/2 cucumber, peeled and cut
- 1/2 bell pepper (red or yellow), cored and diced
- 1/4 red onion, peeled and chopped
- 1 clove garlic, peeled and sliced
- 1/4 cup fresh basil leaves
- 1/4 cup water (optional)
- 1/4 lime, juiced (optional)
- Pinch of sea salt (optional)

<u>INSTRUCTIONS:</u>

1. Wash and prepare all ingredients.
2. Juice the tomato, cucumber, bell pepper, and red onion together.
3. Add garlic, basil leaves, lime juice (if used), and water (if using) to the juicer and process again.
4. Season with sea salt (if using) and mix thoroughly.
5. Chill the juice in the refrigerator for at least 30 minutes before serving.

<u>Tip:</u>

1. This famous Spanish cold soup is rejuvenated and invigorated in juice form.
2. You may modify the spiciness level by adding a pinch of chili flakes or cayenne pepper.

Spirulina Avocado Juice

Prep Time: 5 minutes

Servings: 1

<u>NUTRITIONAL VALUES:</u>

- Calories: 140
- Carbs: 4g
- Sugar: 2g
- Fiber: 3g
- Vitamin C: 2% DV

<u>INGREDIENTS:</u>

- 1/2 avocado, pitted and peeled
- 1/2 cucumber, peeled and cut
- 1 bunch spinach leaves
- 1/2 teaspoon spirulina powder
- 1/4 cup water (optional)
- 1/4 lime, juiced (optional)

1. Wash and prepare all ingredients.
2. Blend the avocado, cucumber, spinach, and spirulina powder together until smooth.
3. Add water (if used) and lime juice (if using) and mix again until fully integrated.
4. Pour into a glass and drink immediately.

Tip:

1. This creamy and green juice is rich with nutritious fats, vitamins, and minerals.
2. The spirulina gives a surge of protein and important minerals.

Refreshing Red Bell Pepper Carrot Juice

Prep Time: 5 minutes

Servings: 1

NUTRITIONAL VALUES:

- Calories: 80
- Carbs: 12g

- Sugar: 8g
- Fiber: 2g
- Vitamin C: 120% DV

INGREDIENTS:

- 1 red bell pepper, cored and diced
- 2 carrots, peeled and sliced
- 1/2 apple, cored and cut
- 1/2 celery stalk, chopped
- 1/4 lime, juiced

INSTRUCTIONS:

1. Wash and prepare all ingredients.
2. Juice the bell pepper, carrots, apple, and celery together.
3. Add lime juice to the juicer and process again.
4. Stir thoroughly and enjoy immediately.

Tip:

1. This colorful juice is naturally sweet and refreshing.
2. The red bell pepper gives a distinct taste and a source of vitamin C.

Spinach Lime Juice

Prep Time: 5 minutes

Servings: 1

NUTRITIONAL VALUES:

- Calories: 60

- Carbs: 5g

- Sugar: 3g

- Fiber: 2g

- Vitamin C: 180% DV

INGREDIENTS:

- 2 handfuls spinach leaves

- 1/2 cucumber, peeled and cut

- 1/2 apple, cored and cut

- 1/4 lime, juiced

- 1/4 cup water (optional)

INSTRUCTIONS:

1. Wash and prepare all ingredients.
2. Juice the cucumber and apple together.
3. Add spinach leaves and lime juice to the juicer and process again.
4. Add water (if using) and whisk thoroughly.
5. Pour into a glass and drink immediately.

Tip:

1. This simple drink is a terrific way to get your daily dose of greens and vitamins.
2. The lime offers a pleasant freshness and helps prevent browning.

Fabulous Fennel Juice Blend

Prep Time: 5 minutes

Servings: 1

NUTRITIONAL VALUES:

- Calories: 80

- Carbs: 15g

- Sugar: 10g

- Fiber: 3g

- Vitamin C: 20% DV

INGREDIENTS:

- 1 fennel bulb, trimmed and chopped

- 1 apple, cored and cut

- 1/2 cucumber, peeled and cut

- 1/4 lemon, juiced

- 1/4 cup water (optional)

INSTRUCTIONS:

1. Wash and prepare all ingredients.
2. Blend the fennel, apple, and cucumber together until smooth.
3. Add lemon juice and water (if using) and mix again until thoroughly integrated.
4. Pour into a glass and drink immediately.

Tip:

1. This earthy and refreshing combination delivers a distinct taste from the fennel.
2. The apple balances the somewhat licorice flavor and the cucumber offers a refreshing impact.
3. Enjoy this juice for a light and healthful treat.

Sweet Potato Power Juice

Prep Time: 5 minutes

Servings: 1

NUTRITIONAL VALUES:

- Calories: 200
- Carbs: 40g
- Sugar: 25g
- Fiber: 4g
- Vitamin A: 300% DV

INGREDIENTS:

- 1 medium sweet potato, peeled and sliced
- 1 carrot, peeled and sliced
- 1/2 apple, cored and cut
- 1/4 ginger root, peeled and diced (optional)
- 1/4 cup almond milk (optional)

INSTRUCTIONS:

1. Wash and prepare all ingredients.
2. Steam or bake the sweet potato until tender (approximately 20-25 minutes).
3. Juice the carrot and apple together.
4. Add the cooked sweet potato and ginger (if using) to the juicer and process again.
5. Add almond milk (if using) and whisk thoroughly.
6. Pour into a glass and drink immediately.

Tip:

1. This creamy and nutritious juice is full with vitamins and minerals, including beta-carotene and potassium.
2. Adding ginger offers a spicy flavor, while almond milk makes a smooth and satisfying texture.

Calming Carrot Juice

Prep Time: 5 minutes

Servings: 1

NUTRITIONAL VALUES:

- Calories: 80
- Carbs: 12g
- Sugar: 8g
- Fiber: 2g
- Vitamin A: 230% DV

INGREDIENTS:

- 2 carrots, peeled and sliced
- 1 apple, cored and cut
- 1/2 cucumber, peeled and cut
- 1/4 celery stalk, chopped
- 1/4 lemon, juiced
- 1 sprig fresh mint (optional)

INSTRUCTIONS:

1. Wash and prepare all ingredients.
2. Juice the carrots, apple, cucumber, and celery together.

3. Add lemon juice and mint (if using) to the juicer and process again.

4. Stir thoroughly and enjoy immediately.

<u>Tip:</u>

1. This calming drink is rich in antioxidants and vitamins, supporting serenity and eye health.

2. The mint offers a refreshing touch, making it suitable for a peaceful time.

Ginger Beet Juice

Prep Time: 5 minutes

Servings: 1

<u>NUTRITIONAL VALUES:</u>

- Calories: 80
- Carbs: 18g
- Sugar: 15g
- Fiber: 2g
- Vitamin C: 20% DV

<u>INGREDIENTS:</u>

- 1 beet, peeled and cut
- 1 carrot, peeled and sliced
- 1/2 apple, cored and cut
- 1/4-inch ginger root, peeled and cut
- 1/4 lime, juiced

<u>INSTRUCTIONS:</u>

1. Wash and prepare all ingredients.

2. Juice the beet, carrot, and apple together.

3. Add ginger and lime juice to the juicer and process again.

4. Stir thoroughly and enjoy immediately.

<u>Tip:</u>

1. This colorful juice mixes the earthy sweetness of beets with the fiery zing of ginger.

2. It's filled with nutrients and delivers a distinct tasting experience.

3. Remember, beets may stain clothes, so be careful when handling them.

Pick-Me-Up Juice Blend

Prep Time: 5 minutes

Servings: 1

<u>NUTRITIONAL VALUES:</u>

- Calories: 130
- Carbs: 25g
- Sugar: 20g
- Fiber: 3g
- Vitamin C: 120% DV

<u>INGREDIENTS:</u>

- 1 bunch spinach leaves
- 1/2 banana, peeled
- 1/2 pineapple, cored and cut
- 1/4 orange, peeled and sliced

- 1/4 cup coconut water

INSTRUCTIONS:

INSTRUCTIONS:

1. Wash and prepare all ingredients.
2. Blend the spinach and banana together until smooth.
3. Add pineapple, orange, and coconut water to the blender and process again until fully incorporated.
4. Pour into a glass and drink immediately.

Tip:

1. This tropical combination is a delightful and refreshing way to gain a surge of energy.
2. The spinach gives minerals, the banana contributes potassium, and the pineapple and orange provide a blast of zesty taste.

Spicy Tomato Juice

Prep Time: 5 minutes

Servings: 1

NUTRITIONAL VALUES:

- Calories: 50
- Carbs: 7g
- Sugar: 5g
- Fiber: 1g
- Vitamin C: 40% DV

INGREDIENTS:

- 2 big tomatoes, cored and cut
- 1/2 celery stalk, chopped
- 1/4 red onion, peeled and chopped (optional)
- 1/4 jalapeño pepper, seeded and chopped (change quantity for desired spice level)
- 1 clove garlic, peeled and sliced
- 1/4 lemon, juiced
- 1/4 teaspoon cayenne pepper (optional)
- Pinch of sea salt
- Pinch of black pepper

INSTRUCTIONS:

1. Wash and prepare all ingredients.
2. Juice the tomatoes, celery, red onion (if using), and jalapeño pepper together.
3. Add garlic, lemon juice, cayenne pepper (if using), salt, and pepper to the juicer and process again.
4. Stir thoroughly and enjoy immediately.

Tip:

1. This homemade spicy tomato juice provides a healthier alternative to store-bought alternatives.
2. Adjust the quantity of jalapeño and cayenne pepper to your chosen degree of spice.
3. For a smoother texture, filter the juice after processing.

Kick-Start Veggie Juice

Prep Time: 5 minutes

Servings: 1

NUTRITIONAL VALUES:

- Calories: 80
- Carbs: 15g
- Sugar: 10g
- Fiber: 3g
- Vitamin C: 120% DV

INGREDIENTS:

- 1 cucumber, peeled and cut
- 1 apple, cored and cut
- 1/2 carrot, peeled and sliced
- 1/2 celery stalk, chopped
- 1/4 lemon, juiced
- 1/4-inch ginger root, peeled and diced (optional)

INSTRUCTIONS:

1. Wash and prepare all ingredients.
2. Juice the cucumber, apple, carrot, and celery together.
3. Add lemon juice and ginger (if using) to the juicer and process again.
4. Stir thoroughly and enjoy immediately.

Tip:

1. This invigorating drink balances sweet and savory ingredients, delivering a pleasant start to your day.
2. The cucumber hydrates, the apple adds sweetness, while the celery and carrot contribute critical vitamins.
3. Customize the ginger quantity for your preferred spicy degree.

Protein Power Juice

Prep Time: 5 minutes

Servings: 1

NUTRITIONAL VALUES:

- Calories: 150
- Carbs: 20g
- Sugar: 15g
- Fiber: 4g
- Protein: 4g

INGREDIENTS:

- 1 bunch spinach leaves
- 1/2 avocado, pitted and peeled
- 1/2 cucumber, peeled and cut
- 1/4 cup unsweetened almond milk
- 1/4 scoop plant-based protein powder (optional)
- 1/4 lime, juiced (optional)

INSTRUCTIONS:

1. Wash and prepare all ingredients.
2. Blend the spinach and avocado until smooth.

3. Add cucumber, almond milk, protein powder (if used), and lime juice (if using) to the blender and process again until completely integrated.

4. Pour into a glass and drink immediately.

<u>Tip:</u>

1. This creamy and protein-rich drink is a great post-workout treat or a quick breakfast choice.

2. The avocado gives healthy fats, the spinach supplies nutrients, and the plant-based protein powder improves satiety.

3. Adjust the ingredients according on your chosen protein amount and taste profile.

Skinny Green Juice

Prep Time: 5 minutes

Servings: 1

NUTRITIONAL VALUES:

- Calories: 60
- Carbs: 5g
- Sugar: 3g
- Fiber: 2g
- Vitamin C: 180% DV

INGREDIENTS:

- 2 handfuls spinach leaves
- 1/2 cucumber, peeled and cut
- 1 celery stalk, chopped
- 1/2 green apple, cored and cut
- 1/4 lemon, juiced

INSTRUCTIONS:

1. Wash and prepare all ingredients.

2. Juice the spinach, cucumber, celery, and apple together.

3. Add lemon juice to the juicer and process again.

4. Stir thoroughly and enjoy immediately.

<u>Tip:</u>

1. This low-calorie and nutrient-rich juice is great for a detoxifying cleanse or a light and refreshing drink.

2. The mix of greens and apple delivers a balanced taste and a boost of vitamins and minerals.

Carrot Celery Cleanse

Prep Time: 5 minutes

Servings: 1

NUTRITIONAL VALUES:

- Calories: 80
- Carbs: 12g
- Sugar: 8g
- Fiber: 3g
- Vitamin A: 230% DV

- 2 carrots, peeled and sliced
- 2 celery stalks, chopped
- 1/2 apple, cored and cut
- 1/4 lemon, juiced
- 1/4-inch ginger root, peeled and diced (optional)

INSTRUCTIONS:

1. Wash and prepare all ingredients.
2. Juice the carrots, celery, and apple together.
3. Add lemon juice and ginger (if using) to the juicer and process again.
4. Stir thoroughly and enjoy immediately.

Tip:

1. This cleaning drink is filled with beta-carotene and antioxidants, aiding good digestion and detoxification.
2. The celery provides natural electrolytes, while the apple balances the taste with a hint of sweetness.
3. Adjust the ginger quantity for your preferred degree of spiciness.

Breakfast of Champions Juice

Prep Time: 5 minutes

Servings: 1

NUTRITIONAL VALUES:

- Calories: 200
- Carbs: 30g
- Sugar: 25g
- Fiber: 4g
- Vitamin C: 140% DV

INGREDIENTS:

- 1/2 banana, frozen and peeled
- 1/4 cup berries (mixed or your favorite), frozen
- 1/4 cup Greek yogurt
- 1/4 cup unsweetened almond milk
- 1/2 scoop plant-based protein powder (optional)
- 1/4 teaspoon chia seeds (optional)

INSTRUCTIONS:

1. Wash and prepare all ingredients.
2. Blend the banana, berries, Greek yogurt, and almond milk together until smooth.
3. Add protein powder (if used) and chia seeds (if using) and mix again until fully integrated.
4. Pour into a glass and drink immediately.

Tip:

1. This protein-packed and creamy juice is a tasty and healthful way to start your day.
2. The frozen banana creates a thick and frosty texture, the berries contribute natural sweetness and antioxidants, and

the Greek yogurt delivers protein and healthy fats.

3. Adjust the ingredients depending on your personal taste and nutritional demands.

Rockin' Radish Juice

Prep Time: 5 minutes

Servings: 1

NUTRITIONAL VALUES:

- Calories: 40
- Carbs: 4g
- Sugar: 2g
- Fiber: 1g
- Vitamin C: 120% DV

INGREDIENTS:

- 1 red radish, trimmed and chopped
- 1 cucumber, peeled and cut
- 1 green apple, cored and cut
- 1/2 celery stalk, chopped
- 1/4 lemon, juiced

INSTRUCTIONS:

1. Wash and prepare all ingredients.
2. Juice the radish, cucumber, apple, and celery together.
3. Add lemon juice to the juicer and process again.
4. Stir thoroughly and enjoy immediately.

Tip:

1. This hot and refreshing juice gives a distinct tasting experience.
2. The radish gives a spicy bite, tempered by the sweetness of the apple and cucumber.
3. The celery gives a cooling effect, making this drink excellent for a hot day.

Green Machine Juice Blend

Prep Time: 5 minutes

Servings: 1

NUTRITIONAL VALUES:

- Calories: 80
- Carbs: 10g
- Sugar: 5g
- Fiber: 4g
- Vitamin C: 180% DV

INGREDIENTS:

- 2 handfuls spinach leaves
- 1/2 cucumber, peeled and cut
- 1 celery stalk, chopped
- 1/2 green bell pepper, cored and cut
- 1/4 lime, juiced
- 1/4-inch ginger root, peeled and diced (optional)

INSTRUCTIONS:

1. Wash and prepare all ingredients.

2. Blend the spinach, cucumber, celery, and bell pepper together until smooth.

3. Add lime juice and ginger (if using) to the blender and pulse again until fully integrated.

4. Pour into a glass and drink immediately.

Tip:

1. This colorful and nutrient-packed combination is a powerhouse of green goodness.

2. The spinach gives iron and minerals, the cucumber hydrates, and the bell pepper adds a hint of sweetness.

3. The ginger delivers a warming kick, increasing the taste and helping digestion.

Red Cabbage Carrot Juice

Prep Time: 5 minutes

Servings: 1

NUTRITIONAL VALUES:

- Calories: 80
- Carbs: 15g
- Sugar: 10g
- Fiber: 2g
- Vitamin C: 50% DV

INGREDIENTS:

- 1/4 red cabbage, cored and chopped
- 2 carrots, peeled and sliced
- 1/2 apple, cored and cut
- 1/4 lemon, juiced

INSTRUCTIONS:

- Wash and prepare all ingredients.
- Juice the red cabbage, carrots, and apple together.
- Add lemon juice to the juicer and process again.
- Stir thoroughly and enjoy immediately.

Tip:

1. This lovely and distinctive juice delivers a brilliant hue and a combination of sweet and slightly sour tastes.

2. The red cabbage is rich in antioxidants, the carrots contribute beta-carotene, and the apple balances the flavor.

3. Enjoy this juice for its nutritional advantages and visual beauty.

Ginger Green Juice Blend

Prep Time: 5 minutes

Servings: 1

NUTRITIONAL VALUES:

- Calories: 70
- Carbs: 10g
- Sugar: 5g

- Fiber: 3g
- Vitamin C: 150% DV

INGREDIENTS:

INGREDIENTS:

- 2 handfuls spinach leaves
- 1/2 cucumber, peeled and cut
- 1 celery stalk, chopped
- 1/2 lime, juiced
- 1/4-inch ginger root, peeled and cut

INSTRUCTIONS:

- Wash and prepare all ingredients.
- Blend the spinach, cucumber, celery, and ginger together until smooth.
- Add lime juice to the blender and process again until fully integrated.
- Pour into a glass and drink immediately.

Tip:

1. This easy and tasty combination is filled with immune-boosting effects.
2. The ginger delivers a warming spice, the spinach supplies iron and vitamins, while the cucumber and celery bring moisture and cooling characteristics.
3. This drink is ideal for a fast pick-me-up or to relieve a sore throat.

Parsley Power Gulp

Prep Time: 5 minutes

Servings: 1

NUTRITIONAL VALUES:

- Calories: 20
- Carbs: 2g
- Sugar: 1g
- Fiber: 1g
- Vitamin C: 130% DV

INGREDIENTS:

- 1 bunch parsley, rinsed and coarsely cut (stems and leaves)
- 1/2 cucumber, peeled and cut
- 1 green apple, cored and cut (optional)
- 1/4 lemon, juiced
- 1/4-inch ginger root, peeled and diced (optional)

INSTRUCTIONS:

1. Wash and prepare all ingredients.
2. Juice the parsley and cucumber together.
3. Add apple (if used), lemon juice, and ginger (if using) to the juicer and process again.
4. Stir thoroughly and enjoy immediately.

Tip:

1. This strong drink offers a punch of vitamins and minerals, including vitamin C and antioxidants. Parsley gives purifying benefits, while the cucumber moisturizes and improves digestion.

2. The added apple balances the taste and ginger provides a spicy bite.

3. Remember, parsley has a strong flavor, so start with a lower quantity and adapt according on your choice.

Liver Detox Tonic

Prep Time: 5 minutes

Servings: 1

NUTRITIONAL VALUES:

- Calories: 90
- Carbs: 15g
- Sugar: 10g
- Fiber: 3g
- Vitamin C: 120% DV

INGREDIENTS:

- 1 beet, peeled and cut
- 2 carrots, peeled and sliced
- 1/2 apple, cored and cut
- 1/4 lemon, juiced
- 1/4-inch ginger root, peeled and diced (optional)
- 1 clove garlic, peeled and diced (optional)

INSTRUCTIONS:

1. Wash and prepare all ingredients.
2. Juice the beet, carrots, and apple together.

3. Add lemon juice, ginger (if used), and garlic (if using) to the juicer and process again.

4. Stir thoroughly and enjoy immediately.

Tip:

1. This earthy and somewhat sweet juice promotes liver health with the cleansing effects of beets and the vitamins and minerals from carrots and apples.

2. The ginger and garlic give a warming kick and further increase the nutritional profile.

3. Remember, beets may stain clothes, so be careful when handling them.

Cucumber Wake-Up Call

Prep Time: 5 minutes

Servings: 1

NUTRITIONAL VALUES:

- Calories: 40
- Carbs: 5g
- Sugar: 2g
- Fiber: 1g
- Vitamin C: 20% DV

INGREDIENTS:

- 2 cucumbers, peeled and cut
- 1 celery stalk, chopped
- 1/2 lime, juiced

- 1/4-inch ginger root, peeled and diced (optional)
- 1 sprig fresh mint (optional)

INSTRUCTIONS:

1. Wash and prepare all ingredients.
2. Juice the cucumbers and celery together.
3. Add lime juice, ginger (if used), and mint (if using) to the juicer and process again.
4. Stir thoroughly and enjoy immediately.

Tip:

1. This delicious and hydrating drink is excellent for a morning pick-me-up.
2. The cucumber cools and hydrates, while the celery provides electrolytes and a delicate taste.
3. The lime juice offers a tart flavor, while the added ginger and mint provide a refreshing twist.

Best Foot Forward Juice

Prep Time: 5 minutes

Servings: 1

NUTRITIONAL VALUES:

- Calories: 80
- Carbs: 12g
- Sugar: 8g
- Fiber: 2g
- Vitamin K: 70% DV

INGREDIENTS:

- 1 handful kale leaves
- 1/2 carrot, peeled and sliced
- 1/2 sweet potato, peeled and sliced
- 1/4 celery stalk, chopped
- 1/4 lemon, juiced

INSTRUCTIONS:

1. Wash and prepare all ingredients.
2. Juice the greens and carrot together.
3. Add sweet potato, celery, and lemon juice to the juicer and process again.
4. Stir thoroughly and enjoy immediately.

Tip:

1. This nutrient-rich juice delivers vitamins, minerals, and antioxidants to assist your physical activities.
2. The kale supplies vitamins K and A, the sweet potato contributes beta-carotene and complex carbs, and the carrot and celery bring numerous beneficial components.
3. Enjoy this juice before or after your exercise for an energy boost and recuperation help.

Minty Mojito Juice

Prep Time: 5 minutes

Servings: 1

NUTRITIONAL VALUES:

- Calories: 80
- Carbs: 15g
- Sugar: 10g
- Fiber: 2g
- Vitamin C: 80% DV

INGREDIENTS:

- 1 bunch spinach leaves
- 1/2 cucumber, peeled and cut
- 1/2 green apple, cored and cut
- 1/4 lime, juiced
- 1 sprig fresh mint
- Pinch of sea salt (optional)

INSTRUCTIONS:

1. Wash and prepare all ingredients.
2. Juice the spinach, cucumber, and apple together.
3. Add lime juice, mint, and salt (if using) to the juicer and process again.
4. Stir thoroughly and enjoy immediately.

Tip:

1. This light and delightful juice puts a spin on the traditional mojito beverage, sans the alcohol.
2. The spinach supplies iron and vitamins, the cucumber hydrates, and the apple balances the taste.
3. The mint offers a cooling and fragrant touch

Cool Cilantro Coconut Juice

Prep Time: 5 minutes

Servings: 1

NUTRITIONAL VALUES:

- Calories: 100
- Carbs: 10g
- Sugar: 8g
- Fiber: 1g
- Vitamin C: 20% DV

INGREDIENTS:

- 1 handful cilantro leaves
- 1/2 cucumber, peeled and cut
- 1/2 green bell pepper, cored and cut
- 1/4 cup unsweetened coconut water
- 1/4 lime, juiced
- Pinch of sea salt (optional)

INSTRUCTIONS:

1. Wash and prepare all ingredients.
2. Juice the cilantro, cucumber, and bell pepper together.
3. Add coconut water, lime juice, and salt (if using) to the juicer and process again.
4. Stir thoroughly and enjoy immediately.

Tip:

1. This tropical-inspired juice delivers a unique flavor combination and a cool, refreshing taste.
2. The cilantro offers a particular flavor and taste, tempered by the sweetness of the bell pepper and the moisturizing characteristics of the cucumber and coconut water.
3. The lime juice gives a tart touch, making this drink excellent for a hot day.

Additional Notes:

- As usual, feel free to alter the ingredients and amounts to your desire.
- For a thicker consistency, add less water or skip it completely.
- If you don't have a juicer, you may combine the ingredients and then filter the mixture through a fine-mesh screen to remove any pulp.
- Remember to wash your veggies and fruits thoroughly before juicing.
- If you have any health problems, talk with your doctor before beginning a juicing plan.
- Enjoy your healthy and tasty vegetable juices!

WEIGHT-LOSS JUICE RECIPES:

Beetroot with Carrot:

Prep Time: 5 minutes

Servings: 1

<u>NUTRITIONAL VALUES:</u>

- Calories: 80
- Carbs: 15g
- Sugar: 10g
- Fiber: 3g
- Vitamin C: 120% DV

<u>INGREDIENTS:</u>

- 1 medium beetroot, peeled and cut
- 2 carrots, peeled and sliced
- 1/2 apple, cored and cut (optional)
- 1/4 lemon, juiced

<u>INSTRUCTIONS:</u>

1. Wash and prepare all ingredients.
2. Juice the beets and carrots together.
3. Add apple (if using) and lemon juice to the juicer and process again.
4. Stir thoroughly and enjoy immediately.

<u>Tip:</u>

1. Beets include nitrates, which may increase blood flow and promote weight control.
2. Carrots give fiber and beta-carotene, supporting satiety and good digestion.

3. Adjust apple quantity for desired sweetness.

Garden Apple and Carrot Juice:

Prep Time: 5 minutes

Servings: 1

<u>NUTRITIONAL VALUES:</u>

- Calories: 80
- Carbs: 12g
- Sugar: 8g
- Fiber: 2g
- Vitamin C: 60% DV

<u>INGREDIENTS:</u>

- 1 bunch spinach leaves
- 1/2 apple, cored and cut
- 1 carrot, peeled and sliced
- 1/2 celery stalk, chopped
- 1/4 lemon, juiced

<u>INSTRUCTIONS:</u>

1. Wash and prepare all ingredients.
2. Juice the spinach and apple together.
3. Add carrot, celery, and lemon juice to the juicer and process again.
4. Stir thoroughly and enjoy immediately.

<u>Tip:</u>

1. Spinach offers iron and vitamins, improving metabolism.
2. Apples include pectin, a fiber that may benefit weight control.
3. Carrots and celery improve hydration and digestion.

Cucumber Protein:

Prep Time: 5 minutes

Servings: 1

<u>NUTRITIONAL VALUES:</u>

- Calories: 60
- Carbs: 5g
- Sugar: 3g
- Fiber: 2g
- Protein: 4g

INGREDIENTS:

- 1 cucumber, peeled and cut
- 1 bunch spinach leaves
- 1/4 avocado, pitted and peeled
- 1/4 cup unsweetened almond milk
- 1/4 scoop plant-based protein powder (optional)

INSTRUCTIONS:

1. Wash and prepare all ingredients.
2. Blend the cucumber and spinach till smooth.
3. Add avocado, almond milk, and protein powder (if using) to the blender and process again until fully incorporated.
4. Pour into a glass and drink immediately.

<u>Tip:</u>

1. Cucumbers are low-calorie and hydrating.
2. Avocados deliver healthful fats and fiber, increasing satiety.
3. Protein powder boosts protein consumption for muscle growth and metabolic assistance.

Apple and Cucumber Juice:

Prep Time: 5 minutes

Servings: 1

<u>NUTRITIONAL VALUES:</u>

- Calories: 60
- Carbs: 10g
- Sugar: 8g
- Fiber: 1g
- Vitamin C: 30% DV

INGREDIENTS:

- 1 apple, cored and cut
- 1 cucumber, peeled and cut
- 1/4 lemon, juiced
- Pinch of ginger root, peeled and diced (optional)

1. Wash and prepare all ingredients.
2. Juice the apple and cucumber together.
3. Add lemon juice and ginger (if using) to the juicer and process again.
4. Stir thoroughly and enjoy immediately.

Tip:

1. Apples give pectin and fiber, boosting satiety.
2. Cucumbers are low-calorie and hydrating.
3. Lemon juice gives a tart taste and improves digestion. Ginger improves metabolism (optional).

Pineapple Juice:

NUTRITIONAL VALUES:

- Calories: 80
- Carbs: 20g
- Sugar: 18g
- Fiber: 1g
- Vitamin C: 130% DV

INGREDIENTS:

- 1 ripe pineapple, peeled and cut

INSTRUCTIONS:

1. Wash and prepare pineapple.
2. Juice the pineapple.
3. Enjoy instantly.

Tip:

1. Pineapple includes bromelain, an enzyme with possible anti-inflammatory properties.
2. Be aware of excessive sugar content.

Watermelon Juice:

NUTRITIONAL VALUES:

- Calories: 60
- Carbs: 15g
- Sugar: 13g
- Fiber: 1g
- Vitamin C: 25% DV

INGREDIENTS:

- 1 slice of seedless watermelon, rind removed

INSTRUCTIONS:

1. Wash and remove the peel from the watermelon slice.
2. Juice the watermelon.
3. Enjoy instantly.

Tip:

1. Watermelon is naturally low in calories and fat but rich in water content, supporting hydration and maybe assisting weight control.
2. Be aware of the sugar content.

Grapefruit Juice:

<u>NUTRITIONAL VALUES:</u>

- Calories: 60
- Carbs: 15g
- Sugar: 9g
- Fiber: 2g
- Vitamin C: 100% DV

<u>INGREDIENTS:</u>

- 1 grapefruit, peeled and sectioned

<u>INSTRUCTIONS:</u>

1. Peel and section the grapefruit.
2. Juice the grapefruit pieces.
3. Enjoy instantly.

<u>Tip:</u>

1. Grapefruit includes naringenin, a chemical with possible weight control advantages.
2. Remember, grapefruit might interfere with some drugs, so check your doctor before ingestion.

Kiwi Juice:

<u>Nutritional Values:</u>

- Calories: 60
- Carbs: 15g
- Sugar: 9g
- Fiber: 2g
- Vitamin C: 260% DV

<u>INGREDIENTS:</u>

- 2 kiwis, peeled and chopped

<u>INSTRUCTIONS:</u>

1. Peel and cut the kiwis.
2. Juice the kiwis.
3. Enjoy instantly.

<u>Tip:</u>

1. Kiwis are rich in fiber and vitamin C, improving digestion and maybe assisting weight control.
2. Be aware of the sugar content.

Minty Fruit Juice:

<u>NUTRITIONAL VALUES:</u>

- Varies based on picked fruits.
- Choose low-sugar choices like berries, melon, etc.

<u>INGREDIENTS:</u>

- Choose a mix of your favorite low-sugar fruits.
- 1 sprig of fresh mint

<u>Optional:</u> 1/4 cup unsweetened almond milk for a creamier texture.

<u>INSTRUCTIONS:</u>

1.   Wash and prepare your selected fruits.

2.   Juice the fruits together with the mint sprig.

3.   Add almond milk (if using) and mix until smooth.

4.   Pour into a glass and drink immediately.

<u>Tip:</u>

1.   This refreshing option allows for customization when utilizing low-sugar fruits.

2.   Mint provides a cooling and perhaps appetite-suppressing impact.

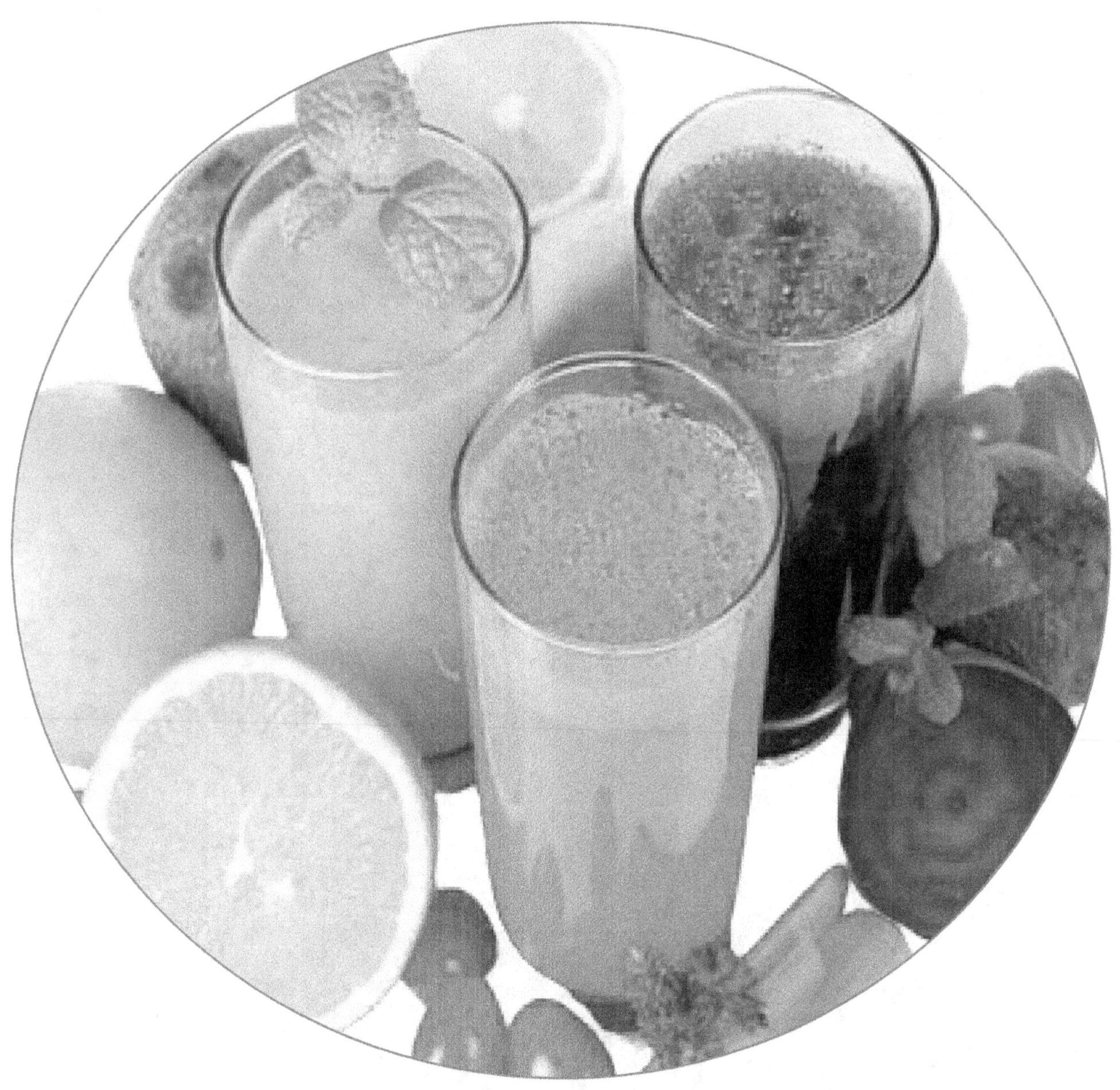

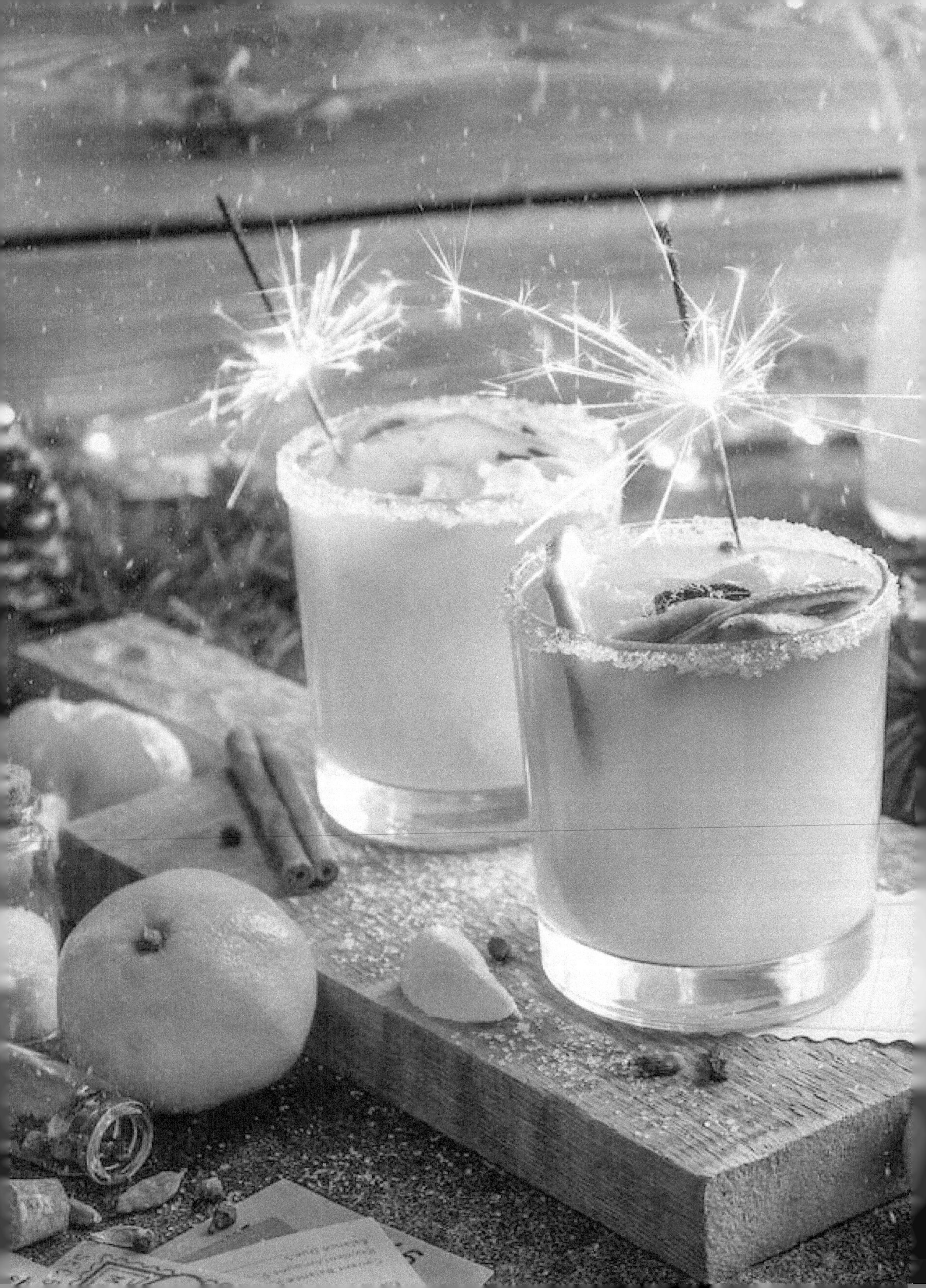

CLEAR AND SMOOTH SKIN JUICE RECIPES:

Strawberry Cherry Juice:

NUTRITIONAL VALUES:

- Calories: 80
- Carbs: 15g
- Sugar: 10g
- Vitamin C: 140% DV

INGREDIENTS:

- 1 handful strawberries, cleaned and hulled
- 1/2 cup cherries, pitted
- 1/2 apple, cored and cut
- 1/4 lemon, juiced

INSTRUCTIONS:

1. Wash and prepare all ingredients.
2. Juice the strawberries, cherries, and apple together.
3. Add lemon juice to the juicer and process again.
4. Stir thoroughly and enjoy immediately.

Tip:

1. Strawberries and cherries give antioxidants and vitamin C, boosting collagen formation and skin health.
2. The apple balances sweetness, while lemon offers a crisp accent.

Apple Carrot Ginger Juice:

NUTRITIONAL VALUES:

- Calories: 80
- Carbs: 15g
- Sugar: 10g
- Vitamin A: 230% DV

INGREDIENTS:

- 1 apple, cored and cut
- 1 carrot, peeled and sliced
- 1/2 cucumber, peeled and sliced (optional)
- 1/4-inch ginger root, peeled and cut

INSTRUCTIONS:

1. Wash and prepare all ingredients.
2. Juice the apple and carrot together.
3. Add cucumber (if using) and ginger to the juicer and process again.
4. Stir thoroughly and enjoy immediately.

Tip:

1. Carrots deliver beta-carotene, encouraging healthy skin cell renewal.
2. Ginger contains anti-inflammatory effects.
3. Cucumber provides hydration (optional).

NUTRITIONAL VALUES:

- Calories: 100
- Carbs: 25g
- Sugar: 20g
- Vitamin C: 60% DV

INGREDIENTS:

- 1 apple, cored and cut
- 1/2 mango, peeled and pitted
- 1/4 lemon, juiced

INSTRUCTIONS:

1. Wash and prepare all ingredients.
2. Juice the apple and mango together.
3. Add lemon juice to the juicer and process again.
4. Stir thoroughly and enjoy immediately.

Tip:

1. Mangoes give vitamins A and C, boosting skin health.
2. The apple balances sweetness, while lemon offers a crisp accent.

Tangy Orange Juice:

NUTRITIONAL VALUES:

- Calories: 60
- Carbs: 15g
- Sugar: 12g

- Vitamin C: 100% DV

INGREDIENTS:

- 1 orange, peeled and sectioned
- 1/2 grapefruit, peeled and sectioned (optional)
- 1/4 lime, juiced

INSTRUCTIONS:

1. Peel and section the orange and grapefruit (if using).
2. Juice the orange and grapefruit (if using) together.
3. Add lime juice to the juicer and process again.
4. Stir thoroughly and enjoy immediately.

Tip:

1. Oranges and grapefruits are rich in vitamin C, crucial for collagen formation and good skin.
2. Adjust grapefruit quantity for desired tartness.

Clearup & Cheerup Juice:

NUTRITIONAL VALUES:

- Calories: 70
- Carbs: 10g
- Sugar: 5g
- Vitamin C: 120% DV

INGREDIENTS:

- 1 bunch spinach leaves
- 1/2 cucumber, peeled and cut
- 1 celery stalk, chopped
- 1/2 apple, cored and cut
- 1/4 lemon, juiced

INSTRUCTIONS:

1. Wash and prepare all ingredients.
2. Juice the spinach, cucumber, celery, and apple together.
3. Add lemon juice to the juicer and process again.
4. Stir thoroughly and enjoy immediately.

Tip:

1. Spinach delivers iron and vitamins, boosting skin health.
2. Cucumber hydrates, and celery gives electrolytes.
3. The apple balances sweetness, and lemon lends a tart accent.

Pineapple Apple Cucumber Refresher:

NUTRITIONAL VALUES:

- Calories: 80
- Carbs: 20g
- Sugar: 15g
- Vitamin C: 80% DV

INGREDIENTS:

- 1/2 pineapple, peeled and cut
- 1/2 apple, cored and cut
- 1/2 cucumber, peeled and cut
- 1/4-inch ginger root, peeled and diced (optional)

INSTRUCTIONS:

1. Wash and prepare all ingredients.
2. Juice the pineapple, apple, and cucumber together.
3. Add ginger (if using) to the juicer and process again.
4. Stir thoroughly and enjoy immediately.

Tip:

1. Pineapple provides bromelain, an enzyme with possible anti-inflammatory properties.
2. The apple balances sweetness, while cucumber provides moisture.
3. Ginger improves metabolism (optional).

Berry Skin Drink:

NUTRITIONAL VALUES:

- Varies based on picked fruit.
- Aim for antioxidant-rich alternatives like blueberries, raspberries, and strawberries.

INGREDIENTS:

- 1 cup mixed berries, washed

- 1/2 cucumber, peeled and sliced (optional)
- 1/4 lemon, juiced

Optional: 1/4 cup unsweetened almond milk for a creamier texture.

1. Wash and prepare berries and cucumber (if using).
2. Juice the berries and cucumber (if using) together.
3. Add lemon juice to the juicer and process again.
4. If using almond milk, combine the juice combination with the milk until smooth.
5. Pour into a glass and drink immediately.

Tip:

1. Berries are rich in antioxidants, boosting skin health.
2. Cucumber provides hydration (optional).
3. Lemon lends a pleasant touch, while almond milk offers extra creaminess (optional).

Skin Cleansing Juice:

NUTRITIONAL VALUES:

- Calories: 40
- Carbs: 5g
- Sugar: 2g

- Vitamin C: 20% DV

INGREDIENTS:

- 1 handful kale leaves
- 1/2 cucumber, peeled and cut
- 1 celery stalk, chopped
- 1/4 green bell pepper, cored and cut
- 1/4 lemon, juiced

INSTRUCTIONS:

1. Wash and prepare all ingredients.
2. Juice the kale, cucumber, celery, and bell pepper together.
3. Add lemon juice to the juicer and process again.
4. Stir thoroughly and enjoy immediately.

Tip:

1. Kale supplies chlorophyll, with possible detoxifying qualities.
2. Cucumber hydrates, and celery gives electrolytes.
3. The bell pepper gives a hint of sweetness, and lemon lends a tart touch.

Green Power Juice:

Prep Time: 5 minutes

Servings: 1

NUTRITIONAL VALUES:

- Calories: 60

- Carbs: 10g

- Sugar: 8g

- Fiber: 3g

- Vitamin C: 120% DV

INGREDIENTS:

- 1 bunch spinach leaves

- 1/2 cucumber, peeled and cut

- 1 celery stalk, chopped

- 1/2 apple, cored and cut

- 1/4-inch ginger root, peeled and diced (optional)

INSTRUCTIONS:

1. Wash and prepare all ingredients.
2. Juice the spinach, cucumber, celery, and apple together.
3. Add ginger (if using) to the juicer and process again.
4. Stir thoroughly and enjoy immediately.

Tip:

1. This nutrient-rich juice delivers vitamins, minerals, and antioxidants to improve general health and perhaps aid to a brighter complexion.

Golden Glow Juice:

Prep Time: 5 minutes

Servings: 1

NUTRITIONAL VALUES:

- Calories: 80

- Carbs: 15g

- Sugar: 12g

- Vitamin C: 100% DV

- Vitamin A: 200% DV

INGREDIENTS:

- 1 carrot, peeled and sliced

- 1/2 pineapple, peeled and cut

- 1/2 orange, peeled and sectioned

- 1/4-inch turmeric root, peeled and diced (optional)

INSTRUCTIONS:

2. Wash and prepare all ingredients.
3. Juice the carrot, pineapple, and orange together.
4. Add turmeric (if used) to the juicer and process again.
5. Stir thoroughly and enjoy immediately.

Tip:

1. This bright juice includes vitamin A from carrots, bromelain from pineapple, and anti-inflammatory curcumin from turmeric, possibly aiding skin health.

Watermelon Mint Cooler:

Prep Time: 5 minutes

Servings: 1

NUTRITIONAL VALUES:

- Calories: 40
- Carbs: 10g
- Sugar: 8g
- Vitamin C: 25% DV

INGREDIENTS:

- 1 cup seedless watermelon chunks
- 1/2 cucumber, peeled and cut
- 5-6 mint leaves
- 1/4 lime, juiced (optional)

INSTRUCTIONS:

2. Wash and prepare all ingredients.
3. Blend the watermelon and cucumber together until smooth.
4. Add mint leaves and lime juice (if using) and mix again until thoroughly integrated.
5. Pour into a glass and drink immediately.

Tip:

1. This delightful combination gives hydration from watermelon and cucumber, while mint adds a cooling and perhaps anti-inflammatory impact.

Berry Chia Smoothie:

Prep Time: 5 minutes

Servings: 1

NUTRITIONAL VALUES:

- Calories: 200
- Carbs: 30g
- Sugar: 20g
- Fiber: 5g
- Vitamin C: 80% DV

INGREDIENTS:

- 1 cup mixed berries (frozen or fresh)
- 1/2 cup unsweetened almond milk
- 1 tbsp. chia seeds
- 1/2 teaspoon honey (optional)

INSTRUCTIONS:

2. Wash and prepare berries (if using fresh).
3. In a blender, mix berries, almond milk, chia seeds, and honey (if using).
4. Blend until smooth and creamy.
5. Pour into a glass and drink immediately.

Tip:

1. This smoothie blends antioxidant-rich berries with chia seeds for fiber and omega-3 fatty acids, perhaps contributing to skin health and general well-being.

ENERGY-BOOSTING AND DE-STRESSING JUICE RECIPES:

Oranges and Cucumber:

Prep Time: 5 minutes

Servings: 1

NUTRITIONAL VALUES:

- Calories: 60
- Carbs: 15g
- Sugar: 12g
- Vitamin C: 100% DV

INGREDIENTS:

- 1 orange, peeled and sectioned
- 1/2 cucumber, peeled and cut

INSTRUCTIONS:

2. Wash and prepare all ingredients.
3. Juice the orange and cucumber together.
4. Stir thoroughly and enjoy immediately.

Tip:

1. This delicious beverage contains vitamin C from oranges and hydration from cucumber, encouraging alertness and maybe reducing weariness.

Apple and Cucumber:

Prep Time: 5 minutes

Servings: 1

NUTRITIONAL VALUES:

- Calories: 60
- Carbs: 15g
- Sugar: 10g
- Fiber: 2g
- Vitamin C: 30% DV

INGREDIENTS:

- 1 apple, cored and cut
- 1/2 cucumber, peeled and cut
- 1/4 lemon, juiced (optional)

INSTRUCTIONS:

2. Wash and prepare all ingredients.
3. Juice the apple and cucumber together.
4. Add lemon juice (if used) to the juicer and process again.
5. Stir thoroughly and enjoy immediately.

Tip:

1. This stimulating beverage delivers natural sugars from apples and moisture from cucumber, while lemon gives a zesty punch (optional).

Cucumber and Tomato:

Prep Time: 5 minutes

Servings: 1

NUTRITIONAL VALUES:

- Calories: 40
- Carbs: 8g
- Sugar: 4g
- Vitamin C: 25% DV
- Lycopene (from tomatoes)

INGREDIENTS:

- 1 cucumber, peeled and cut
- 1 tomato, cored and cut
- 1/4 lime, juiced (optional)

INSTRUCTIONS:

1. Wash and prepare all ingredients.
2. Juice the cucumber and tomato together.
3. Add lime juice (if used) to the juicer and process again.
4. Stir thoroughly and enjoy immediately.

Tip:

1. This hydrated drink mixes cucumber and tomato, delivering electrolytes and lycopene, an antioxidant possibly assisting stress management.

Carrot and Cucumber:

Prep Time: 5 minutes

Servings: 1

NUTRITIONAL VALUES:

- Calories: 60
- Carbs: 10g
- Sugar: 8g
- Vitamin A: 230% DV (from carrots)

INGREDIENTS:

- 1 carrot, peeled and sliced
- 1 cucumber, peeled and cut
- 1/4-inch ginger root, peeled and diced (optional)

INSTRUCTIONS:

1. Wash and prepare all ingredients.
2. Juice the carrot and cucumber together.
3. Add ginger (if using) to the juicer and process again.
4. Stir thoroughly and enjoy immediately.

Tip:

1. This bright juice delivers beta-carotene from carrots and moisture from cucumber, encouraging energy and maybe supporting a healthy immune system.

Celery, Onion, Tomato Juice:

Prep Time: 5 minutes

Servings: 1

- Calories: 40
- Carbs: 8g
- Sugar: 4g
- Vitamin C: 20% DV

INGREDIENTS:

- 2 celery stalks, chopped
- 1/4 red onion, peeled and chopped
- 1 tomato, cored and cut

INSTRUCTIONS:

1. Wash and prepare all ingredients.
2. Juice the celery, onion, and tomato together.
3. Stir thoroughly and enjoy immediately.

Tip:

1. This savory juice contains electrolytes from celery and vitamin C from tomato, perhaps helping hydration and alertness.

Broccoli:

Prep Time: 5 minutes

Servings: 1

NUTRITIONAL VALUES:

- Calories: 30
- Carbs: 5g
- Sugar: 2g
- Vitamin C: 80% DV
- Sulforaphane (from broccoli)

INGREDIENTS:

- 1 cup broccoli florets (steamed or blanched)
- 1/2 apple, cored and cut
- 1/4 lemon, juiced

INSTRUCTIONS:

1. Steam or blanch the broccoli florets until tender.
2. Wash and prepare the apple and lemon.
3. Blend the steamed/blanched broccoli, apple, and lemon juice together until smooth.
4. Strain the combined mixture through a cheesecloth or fine-mesh sieve to remove any pulp.
5. Enjoy instantly.

Tip:

1. This unusual drink combines vitamin C and sulforaphane, a chemical found in broccoli with possible advantages for energy and well-being.
2. The apple provides sweetness, while lemon offers a cooling touch.

Carrot Pepper Juice:

Prep Time: 5 minutes

Servings: 1

NUTRITIONAL VALUES:

- Calories: 60
- Carbs: 12g
- Sugar: 8g
- Vitamin A: 200% DV (from carrots)
- Vitamin C: 60% DV (from bell peppers)

Prep Time: 5 minutes

Servings: 1

NUTRITIONAL VALUES:

- Calories: 100
- Carbs: 25g
- Sugar: 20g
- Fiber: 4g
- Vitamin C: 40% DV

INGREDIENTS:

- 1 carrot, peeled and sliced
- 1/2 bell pepper, cored and cut
- 1/2 cucumber, peeled and sliced (optional)
- 1/4 inch ginger root, peeled and diced (optional)

INGREDIENTS:

- 1 apple, cored and cut
- 1 Asian pear, cored and cut
- 1/2 handful spinach leaves
- 1/4 cucumber, peeled and diced (optional)
- 1/4 lemon, juiced (optional)

INSTRUCTIONS:

1. Wash and prepare all ingredients.
2. Juice the carrot and bell pepper together.
3. Add cucumber (if used) and ginger (if using) to the juicer and process again.
4. Stir thoroughly and enjoy immediately.

INSTRUCTIONS:

1. Wash and prepare all ingredients.
2. Blend the apple, Asian pear, and spinach leaves until smooth.
3. Add cucumber (if used) and lemon juice (if using) to the blender and process again until thoroughly integrated.
4. Pour into a glass and drink immediately.

Tip:

1. This colorful juice contains beta-carotene from carrots and vitamin C from bell peppers, delivering possible energy-boosting and immune-supporting benefits.
2. Cucumber and ginger give moisture and a bit of spiciness (optional).

Tip:

1. This combination blends natural sugars from fruits with fiber from spinach,

delivering continuous energy and possible digestive advantages.

2. Cucumber offers moisture (optional), and lemon lends a tart touch (optional).

Watermelon - Mint Juice:

Prep Time: 5 minutes

Servings: 1

NUTRITIONAL VALUES:

- Calories: 60
- Carbs: 15g
- Sugar: 13g
- Vitamin C: 25% DV

INGREDIENTS:

- 1 cup seedless watermelon chunks
- 5-6 mint leaves
- 1/4 lime, juiced (optional)

INSTRUCTIONS:

1. Wash and prepare all ingredients.
2. Juice the watermelon until smooth.
3. Add mint leaves and lime juice (if using) to the juicer and process again.
4. Stir thoroughly and enjoy immediately.

Tip:

1. This delicious beverage combines natural sugars from watermelon and

hydration, increasing alertness and reducing weariness.

2. Mint gives a cooling and relaxing effect.

Green Grapes Juice:

Prep Time: 5 minutes

Servings: 1

NUTRITIONAL VALUES:

- Calories: 60
- Carbs: 15g
- Sugar: 12g
- Vitamin C: 15% DV

INGREDIENTS:

- 1 cup green grapes, washed and stemmed

INSTRUCTIONS:

1. Wash and prepare the green grapes.
2. Juice the grapes.
3. Stir thoroughly and enjoy immediately.

Tip:

1. This simple drink contains natural sugars from grapes, offering instantly accessible energy.
2. While weaker in vitamins and minerals compared to other alternatives, it might be a fast and refreshing choice.

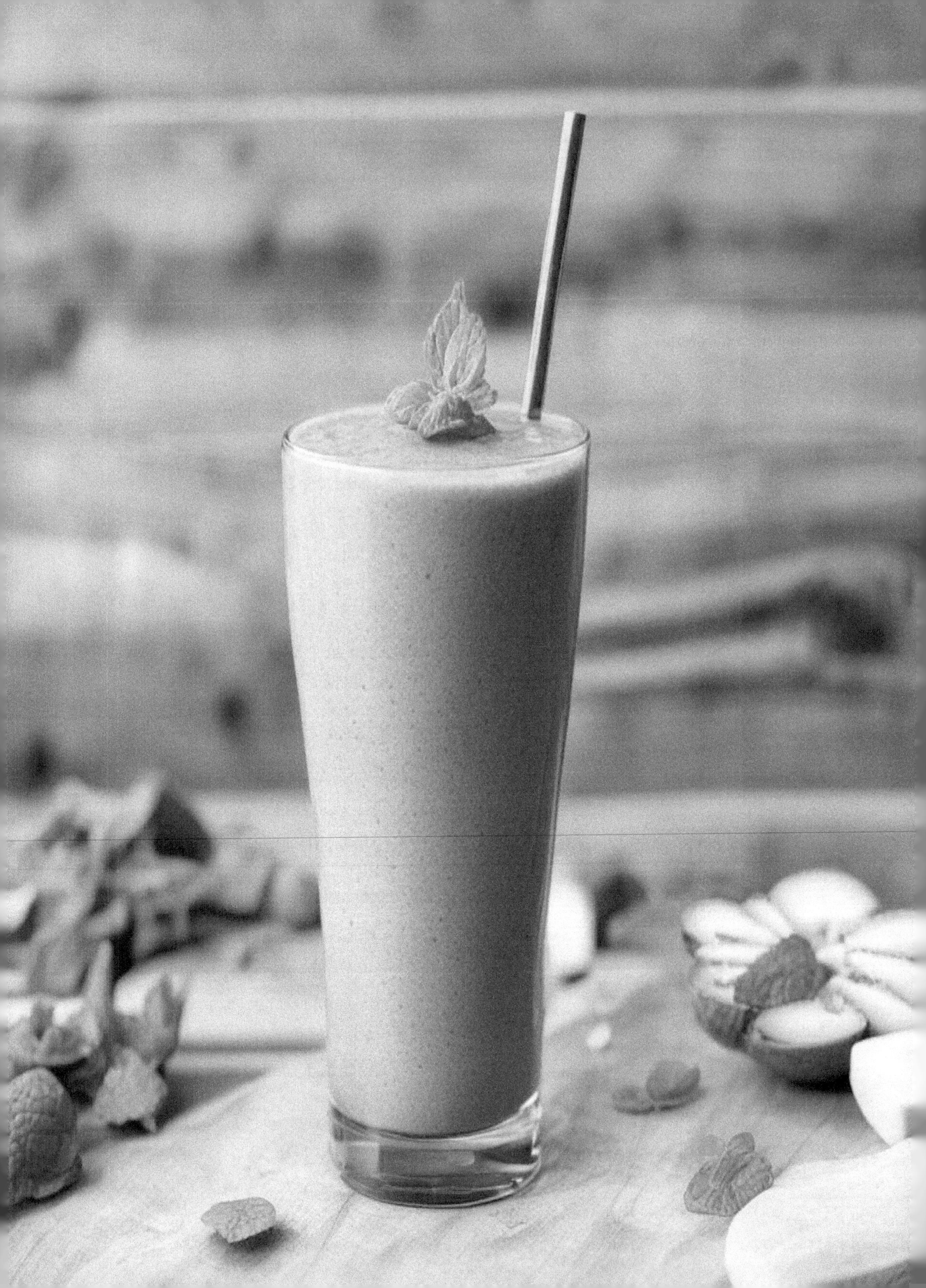

GREEN JUICE RECIPES:

Green Goodness Juice:

For: Hydration and general well-being

Prep Time: 5 minutes

Servings: 1

NUTRITIONAL VALUES:

- Calories: 60
- Carbs: 10g
- Sugar: 8g
- Fiber: 3g
- Vitamin C: 120% DV

INGREDIENTS:

- 1 bunch spinach leaves
- 1/2 cucumber, peeled and cut
- 1 celery stalk, chopped
- 1/2 apple, cored and cut
- 1/4 lemon, juiced

INSTRUCTIONS:

1. Wash and prepare all ingredients.
2. Juice the spinach, cucumber, celery, and apple together.
3. Add lemon juice to the juicer and process again.
4. Stir thoroughly and enjoy immediately.

Tip:

1. This multipurpose drink contains vitamins, minerals, and antioxidants from diverse sources, increasing hydration and supporting general health.

Glorious Green Juice:

For: Energy and detoxification (potential)

Prep Time: 5 minutes

Servings: 1

NUTRITIONAL VALUES:

- Calories: 80
- Carbs: 15g
- Sugar: 12g
- Fiber: 4g
- Vitamin C: 80% DV

INGREDIENTS:

- 1 handful kale leaves
- 1/2 cucumber, peeled and cut
- 1 celery stalk, chopped
- 1/2 green bell pepper, cored and cut
- 1/4-inch ginger root, peeled and diced (optional)

INSTRUCTIONS:

1. Wash and prepare all ingredients.
2. Juice the kale, cucumber, celery, and bell pepper together.
3. Add ginger (if using) to the juicer and process again.

4. Stir thoroughly and enjoy immediately.

Tip:

1. This colorful drink blends kale's chlorophyll with antioxidants from bell pepper and ginger (optional), perhaps increasing energy levels and detoxification processes.

Beautiful Beet Juice:

For: Skin health and possibly anti-inflammatory properties

Prep Time: 5 minutes

Servings: 1

NUTRITIONAL VALUES:

- Calories: 80
- Carbs: 18g
- Sugar: 15g
- Fiber: 2g
- Vitamin C: 20% DV
- Nitrates (from beets)

INGREDIENTS:

- 1/2 medium beet, peeled and sliced
- 1 carrot, peeled and sliced
- 1 apple, cored and cut
- 1/4 lemon, juiced

INSTRUCTIONS:

1. Wash and prepare all ingredients.

2. Juice the beet, carrot, and apple together.

3. Add lemon juice to the juicer and process again.

4. Stir thoroughly and enjoy immediately.

Tip:

1. Beets give nitrates, perhaps promoting blood flow and skin health.

2. This drink blends them with vitamins and antioxidants from carrots and apples.

Green Good Morning Juice:

For: Digestive support and a pleasant start to the day

Prep Time: 5 minutes

Servings: 1

NUTRITIONAL VALUES:

- Calories: 40
- Carbs: 8g
- Sugar: 4g
- Fiber: 3g
- Vitamin C: 25% DV

INGREDIENTS:

- 1 bunch spinach leaves
- 1/2 cucumber, peeled and cut
- 1 celery stalk, chopped
- 1/2 green apple, cored and cut

* 1/4-inch ginger root, peeled and diced (optional)

INSTRUCTIONS:

1. Wash and prepare all ingredients.
2. Juice the spinach, cucumber, celery, and apple together.
3. Add ginger (if using) to the juicer and process again.
4. Stir thoroughly and enjoy immediately.

Tip:

1. This light and delicious drink blends digestive-supporting components like ginger (optional) with hydrating cucumber and vitamins from spinach and apple.

Seven-Layer Green Juice:

For: Variety and a concentrated dose of nutrients

Prep Time: 10 minutes

Servings: 1

NUTRITIONAL VALUES:

* Varies based on selected components.
* Aim for a varied mix of nutrient-rich greens and possible extras.

INGREDIENTS:

Choose 7 different green leafy greens and veggies such as:

* Spinach
* Kale
* Romaine lettuce
* Celery
* Cucumber
* Green bell pepper
* Broccoli florets

INSTRUCTIONS:

2. Wash and prepare all components carefully.
3. Layer your selected ingredients one by one into the juicer's feed tube. Start with the tougher veggies like celery and work your way up to softer greens like spinach.
4. Juice each layer gently, enabling the juicer to obtain optimum nutrients.
5. If desired, add alternative items like ginger, lemon juice, or apple for enhanced taste or nutrition.
6. Stir thoroughly and enjoy immediately.

Tips:

1. This recipe allows you creativity and customization.
2. Experiment with various mixes of greens and veggies to discover your favorite mixture.

3. Start with lower amounts of strong-flavored ingredients like kale or ginger and adapt to your taste preference.

4. If using a centrifugal juicer, try filtering the juice through a cheesecloth for a smoother consistency.

5. Remember, although green juices may be a healthy supplement to your diet, they should not replace a balanced meal.

6. Consult a healthcare professional before making substantial dietary changes.

Additional Green Juice Notes:

Bitter Taste: Some green juices may have a bitter taste owing to substances like chlorophyll. Adding fruits like apple or pear might help temper the bitterness.

Oxalates: Certain plants like spinach and beets contain oxalates, which may bind to calcium and possibly interfere with its absorption. If you have kidney difficulties, see a healthcare practitioner before ingesting big quantities of these veggies.

Fiber: Juicing eliminates much of the fiber from fruits and vegetables. While this might make the juice simpler to digest, it also diminishes its fiber content. Consider integrating entire fruits and veggies in your diet with juicing for a more balanced fiber intake.

Dreamy Green Juice:

For: Relaxation and possibly sleep assistance

Prep Time: 5 minutes

Servings: 1

NUTRITIONAL VALUES:

- Calories: 60
- Carbs: 10g
- Sugar: 8g
- Fiber: 3g
- Vitamin C: 80% DV
- Magnesium (from romaine lettuce)

INGREDIENTS:

- 1 handful romaine lettuce leaves
- 1/2 cucumber, peeled and cut
- 1 celery stalk, chopped
- 1/2 banana, frozen (optional)
- 1/4 avocado, peeled and pitted (optional)
- 1/4 lemon, juiced

INSTRUCTIONS:

1. Wash and prepare all ingredients.
2. Juice the romaine lettuce, cucumber, and celery together.
3. Add banana (if used), avocado (if using), and lemon juice to the juicer and process again.
4. Stir thoroughly and enjoy immediately.

Tip:

1. This creamy and possibly sleep-supportive drink mixes romaine lettuce for magnesium, banana for potassium, and avocado for healthy fats (optional).

2. Enjoy chilled for an added relaxing effect.

Spicy Green Juice:

For: A delicious and invigorating kick

Prep Time: 5 minutes

Servings: 1

NUTRITIONAL VALUES:

- Calories: 50
- Carbs: 8g
- Sugar: 4g
- Fiber: 2g
- Vitamin C: 20% DV

INGREDIENTS:

- 1 bunch spinach leaves
- 1/2 cucumber, peeled and cut
- 1 celery stalk, chopped
- 1/2 jalapeño pepper, seeded and chopped (according to your spice desire)
- 1/4 lime, juiced
- 1/4-inch ginger root, peeled and diced (optional)

INSTRUCTIONS:

1. Wash and prepare all ingredients.

2. Juice the spinach, cucumber, celery, and jalapeño together.

3. Add ginger (if used) and lime juice to the juicer and process again.

4. Stir thoroughly and enjoy immediately.

Tip:

1. This drink delivers a spicy and invigorating combination with vitamin C from spinach and a kick from jalapeño.

2. Adjust the pepper quantity to your spicy tolerance.

Mango Tango Green Juice:

For: A tropical touch on green juice

Prep Time: 5 minutes

Servings: 1

NUTRITIONAL VALUES:

- Calories: 80
- Carbs: 18g
- Sugar: 15g
- Fiber: 2g
- Vitamin C: 100% DV

INGREDIENTS:

- 1 handful kale leaves
- 1/2 cucumber, peeled and cut
- 1 celery stalk, chopped
- 1/2 mango, peeled and pitted

- 1/4 lime, juiced

INSTRUCTIONS:

1. Wash and prepare all ingredients.
2. Juice the kale, cucumber, and celery together.
3. Add mango and lime juice to the juicer and process again.
4. Stir thoroughly and enjoy immediately.

Tip:

1. This colorful juice mixes the sweetness of mango with the benefits of kale, delivering a pleasant and vitamin-rich choice.

Brilliant Brussels Juice:

For: A unique and nutrient-packed combination

Prep Time: 5 minutes

Servings: 1

NUTRITIONAL VALUES:

- Calories: 60
- Carbs: 10g
- Sugar: 5g
- Fiber: 4g
- Vitamin K: 100% DV (from Brussels sprouts)

INGREDIENTS:

- 1 bunch Brussels sprouts, cut and halved
- 1/2 cucumber, peeled and cut
- 1 celery stalk, chopped
- 1/2 green apple, cored and cut
- 1/4 lemon, juiced

INSTRUCTIONS:

1. Wash and prepare all ingredients.
2. Juice the Brussels sprouts, cucumber, and celery together.
3. Add apple and lemon juice to the juicer and process again.
4. Stir thoroughly and enjoy immediately.

Tip:

1. This unusual drink delivers vitamin K from Brussels sprouts, antioxidants from green apple, and hydration from cucumber.
2. Its mildly spicy taste could need getting accustomed to.

Double Trouble Broccoli Juice:

For: A concentrated dosage of minerals and possibly detox help

Prep Time: 5 minutes

Servings: 1

NUTRITIONAL VALUES:

- Calories: 40
- Carbs: 5g

- Sugar: 2g
- Vitamin C: 80% DV
- Sulforaphane (from broccoli)

- 1 cup broccoli florets (steamed or blanched)
- 1/2 green apple, cored and cut
- 1/4 lemon, juiced

INSTRUCTIONS:

1. Steam or blanch the broccoli florets until tender.
2. Wash and prepare the apple and lemon.
3. Blend the steamed/blanched broccoli, apple, and lemon juice together until smooth.
4. Strain the combined mixture through a cheesecloth or fine-mesh sieve to remove any pulp.
5. Enjoy instantly.

Tip:

1. This unusual drink combines concentrated fiber and minerals from broccoli, coupled with vitamin C from the apple and lemon.
2. It could have a little earthy flavor because to the broccoli, but the apple helps balance it out.

Merry Melon Dream Juice:

For: A nourishing and refreshing green juice with a sweet twist

Prep Time: 5 minutes

Servings: 1

NUTRITIONAL VALUES:

- Calories: 60
- Carbs: 15g
- Sugar: 12g
- Vitamin C: 100% DV (from cantaloupe)

INGREDIENTS:

- 1 bunch spinach leaves
- 1/2 cucumber, peeled and chopped
- 1 celery stalk, chopped
- 1/2 cantaloupe melon, peeled and seeded
- 1/4 lime, juiced

INSTRUCTIONS:

1. Wash and prepare all ingredients.
2. Juice the spinach, cucumber, and celery together.
3. Add cantaloupe and lime juice to the juicer and process again.
4. Stir thoroughly and enjoy immediately.

Tip:

1. This colorful juice blends the sweetness of cantaloupe with the benefits of

spinach, delivering a hydrated and refreshing choice.

Sensibly Sweet Juice:

For: A balanced green juice with mild sweetness

Prep Time: 5 minutes

Servings: 1

<u>NUTRITIONAL VALUES:</u>

- Calories: 50
- Carbs: 8g
- Sugar: 4g
- Fiber: 3g
- Vitamin C: 80% DV

<u>INGREDIENTS:</u>

- 1 handful kale leaves
- 1/2 cucumber, peeled and chopped
- 1 celery stalk, chopped 1/2 green apple, cored and chopped
- 1/4 lemon, juiced

<u>INSTRUCTIONS:</u>

1. Wash and prepare all ingredients.
2. Juice the kale, cucumber, and celery together.
3. Add apple and lemon juice to the juicer and process again.
4. Stir thoroughly and enjoy immediately.

<u>Tip:</u>

1. This juice delivers a mix of sweetness from the apple and acidity from the lemon, while retaining a reduced sugar level compared to choices containing melons.

Tossed Salad Juice:

For: A diversified and nutrient-rich green juice combination

Prep Time: 5 minutes

Servings: 1

<u>NUTRITIONAL VALUES:</u>

- Varies based on selected components.
- Aim for a varied range of nutrient-rich greens and veggies.

<u>INGREDIENTS:</u>

- Choose at least 5 different green leafy vegetables and veggies such as:
- Spinach
- Kale
- Romaine lettuce
- Celery
- Cucumber
- Green bell pepper
- Broccoli florets
- Carrots (optional)

<u>INSTRUCTIONS:</u>

1. Wash and prepare all components carefully.

2. Layer your selected ingredients one by one into the juicer's feed tube. Start with the tougher veggies like celery and work your way up to softer greens like spinach.

3. Juice each layer gently, enabling the juicer to obtain optimum nutrients.

4. If desired, add alternative items like ginger, lemon juice, or apple for enhanced taste or nutrition.

5. Stir thoroughly and enjoy immediately.

Tip:

1. This recipe allows for creativity and customization.

2. Experiment with various mixes of greens and veggies to discover your favorite mixture.

Cool Cauliflower Juice:

For: A light and pleasant green juice with a distinctive touch

Prep Time: 5 minutes

Servings: 1

NUTRITIONAL VALUES:

- Calories: 40
- Carbs: 5g
- Sugar: 2g

- Vitamin C: 50% DV
- Choline (from cauliflower)

INGREDIENTS:

- 1 handful romaine lettuce leaves
- 1/2 cucumber, peeled and cut
- 1/2 cup cauliflower florets
- 1/4 lime, juiced
- 1/4-inch ginger root, peeled and diced (optional)

INSTRUCTIONS:

1. Wash and prepare all ingredients.

2. Juice the romaine lettuce and cucumber together.

3. Add cauliflower, lime juice, and ginger (if using) to the juicer and process again.

4. Stir thoroughly and enjoy immediately.

Tip:

1. This juice delivers a distinct and light taste with the inclusion of cauliflower.

2. Ginger (optional) provides a touch of warmth.

Refreshing Green Juice:

For: A traditional and hydrating green juice

Prep Time: 5 minutes

Servings: 1

NUTRITIONAL VALUES:

- Calories: 50
- Carbs: 8g
- Sugar: 4g
- Fiber: 3g
- Vitamin C: 70% DV (approximate)

INGREDIENTS:

- 1 bunch spinach leaves
- 1/2 cucumber, peeled and chopped
- 1 celery stalk, chopped
- 1/2 green apple, cored and chopped
- 1/4 lemon, juiced

INSTRUCTIONS:

1. Wash and prepare all ingredients.
2. Juice the spinach, cucumber, and celery together.
3. Add apple and lemon juice to the juicer and process again.
4. Stir thoroughly and enjoy immediately.

Tip:

1. This traditional green juice delivers an excellent combination of sweetness from the apple and acidity from the lemon, delivering hydration and important vitamins.

Tropical Twist Green Juice:

For: A pleasant and tasty spin on the basic green juice

Prep Time: 5 minutes

Servings: 1

NUTRITIONAL VALUES:

- Calories: 70
- Carbs: 15g
- Sugar: 12g
- Fiber: 2g
- Vitamin C: 120% DV (approximate)

INGREDIENTS:

- 1 bunch spinach leaves
- 1/2 cucumber, peeled and chopped
- 1 celery stalk, chopped
- 1/2 mango, peeled and pitted
- 1/4 lime, juiced

INSTRUCTIONS:

2. Wash and prepare all ingredients.
3. Juice the spinach, cucumber, and celery together.
4. Add mango and lime juice to the juicer and process again.
5. Stir thoroughly and enjoy immediately.

Tip:

1. This variant adds the sweetness and tropical taste of mango, making it a wonderful and refreshing alternative.

For: A powerful dose of green nourishment

Prep Time: 5 minutes

Servings: 1

NUTRITIONAL VALUES:

- Calories: 60
- Carbs: 10g
- Sugar: 5g
- Fiber: 4g
- Vitamin A: 200% DV (from kale)

INGREDIENTS:

- 1 handful kale leaves
- 1 bunch spinach leaves
- 1/2 romaine lettuce leaves
- 1/2 cucumber, peeled and chopped
- 1 celery stalk, chopped
- 1/4 lemon, juiced

INSTRUCTIONS:

2. Wash and prepare all ingredients.
3. Juice the kale, spinach, and romaine lettuce together.
4. Add cucumber, celery, and lemon juice to the juicer and process again.
5. Stir thoroughly and enjoy immediately.

Tip:

1. This drink includes diverse dark leafy greens for their concentrated vitamins and minerals, delivering a significant nutritious boost.

For: An invigorating green juice with a kick

Prep Time: 5 minutes

Servings: 1

NUTRITIONAL VALUES:

- Calories: 80
- Carbs: 15g
- Sugar: 12g
- Fiber: 3g
- Vitamin C: 100% DV

INGREDIENTS:

- 1 bunch spinach leaves
- 1/2 cucumber, peeled and chopped
- 1 celery stalk, chopped
- 1/2 green apple, cored and chopped
- 1/4-inch ginger root, peeled and chopped
- 1/4 lemon, juiced

INSTRUCTIONS:

1. Wash and prepare all ingredients.
2. Juice the spinach, cucumber, and celery together.
3. Add apple, ginger, and lemon juice to the juicer and process again.
4. Stir thoroughly and enjoy immediately.

1. This drink blends natural sugars from the apple with the stimulating characteristics of ginger for an energy boost.

2. Adjust the ginger quantity to your spicy preference.

Jolly Green Giant Juice:

For: A pleasant and tasty green juice with extra sweetness

Prep Time: 5 minutes

Servings: 1

NUTRITIONAL VALUES:

- Calories: 80
- Carbs: 20g
- Sugar: 18g
- Fiber: 2g
- Vitamin C: 70% DV

INGREDIENTS:

- 1 bunch spinach leaves
- 1/2 cucumber, peeled and cut
- 1 celery stalk, chopped
- 1/2 pear, cored and cut
- 1/4 pineapple, chopped (peeled if preferred)
- 1/4 lime, juiced

INSTRUCTIONS:

1. Wash and prepare all ingredients.
2. Juice the spinach, cucumber, and celery together.
3. Add pear, pineapple, and lime juice to the juicer and process again.
4. Stir thoroughly and enjoy immediately.

Tip:

1. This juice mixes the sweetness of pear and pineapple with the benefits of green components, making it a delightful and refreshing alternative.

Beets Me Blend:

For: A unusual and possibly cleansing green juice

Prep Time: 5 minutes

Servings: 1

NUTRITIONAL VALUES:

- Calories: 80
- Carbs: 18g
- Sugar: 15g
- Fiber: 4g Nitrates (from beets)

INGREDIENTS:

- 1 handful kale leaves
- 1/2 cucumber, peeled and chopped
- 1 celery stalk, chopped
- 1/2 beet, peeled and chopped
- 1/2 green apple, cored and chopped

- 1/4 lemon, juiced

1. Wash and prepare all ingredients.
2. Juice the kale, cucumber, celery, and beet together.
3. Add apple and lemon juice to the juicer and process again.
4. Stir thoroughly and enjoy immediately.

Tip:

1. This drink mixes beets for their possible detoxifying effects and nitrates with the advantages of other green components.
2. It could have a little earthy flavor because to the beets.

Simply Sweet Green Juice:

For: A gently sweetened and pleasant green juice

Prep Time: 5 minutes

Servings: 1

NUTRITIONAL VALUES:

- Calories: 50
- Carbs: 8g
- Sugar: 5g
- Fiber: 3g
- Vitamin C: 50% DV (approximate)

INGREDIENTS:

- 1 bunch spinach leaves
- 1/2 cucumber, peeled and chopped
- 1 celery stalk, chopped
- 1/4 green apple, cored and chopped
- 1/4 pear, cored and chopped
- 1/4 lime, juiced (optional)

INSTRUCTIONS:

1. Wash and prepare all ingredients.
2. Juice the spinach, cucumber, and celery together.
3. Add apple, pear, and lime juice (if used) to the juicer and process again.
4. Stir thoroughly and enjoy immediately.

Tip:

1. This juice gives a mild sweetness from the pear and apple, making it delightful without overpowering sweetness.
2. Adding lime juice (optional) provides a delightful tang.

Lean, Mean Green Juice:

For: A low-calorie green juice filled with nutrients

Prep Time: 5 minutes

Servings: 1

NUTRITIONAL VALUES:

- Calories: 40
- Carbs: 5g

- Sugar: 2g
- Fiber: 3g
- Vitamin C: 70% DV (approximate)

INGREDIENTS:

- 1 handful romaine lettuce leaves
- 1/2 cucumber, peeled and chopped
- 1 celery stalk, chopped
- 1/4 green bell pepper, cored and chopped
- 1/4 lemon, juiced

INSTRUCTIONS:

1. Wash and prepare all ingredients.
2. Juice the romaine lettuce, cucumber, celery, and bell pepper together.
3. Add lemon juice to the juicer and process again.
4. Stir thoroughly and enjoy immediately.

Tip:

1. This juice combines romaine lettuce and green bell pepper for decreased sugar content while keeping critical vitamins and minerals.
2. It delivers a pleasant and mild taste.

INDEX RECIPE

A

B

C

D

E

F

G

H

J

K

L

M

O

P

R

S

T

V

W

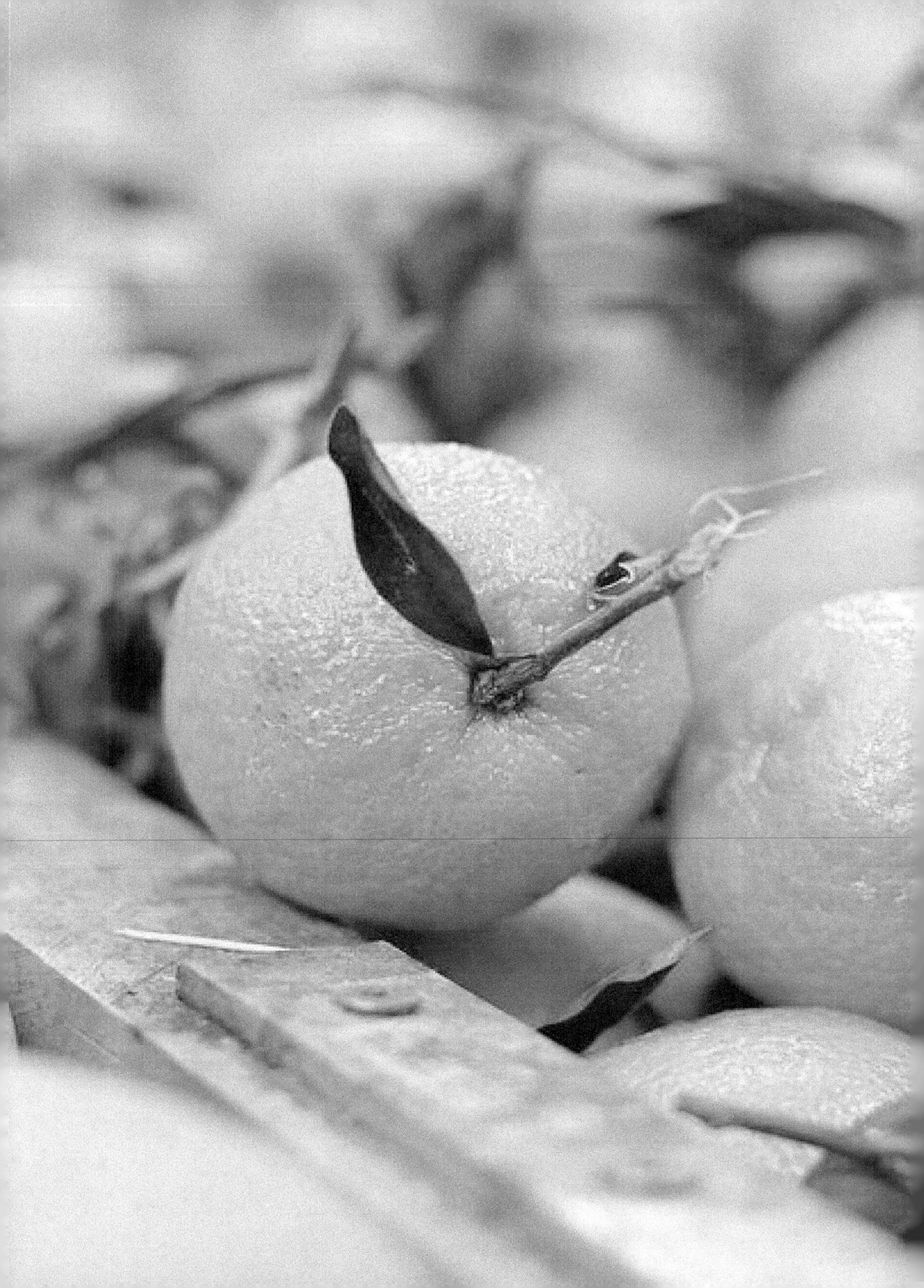

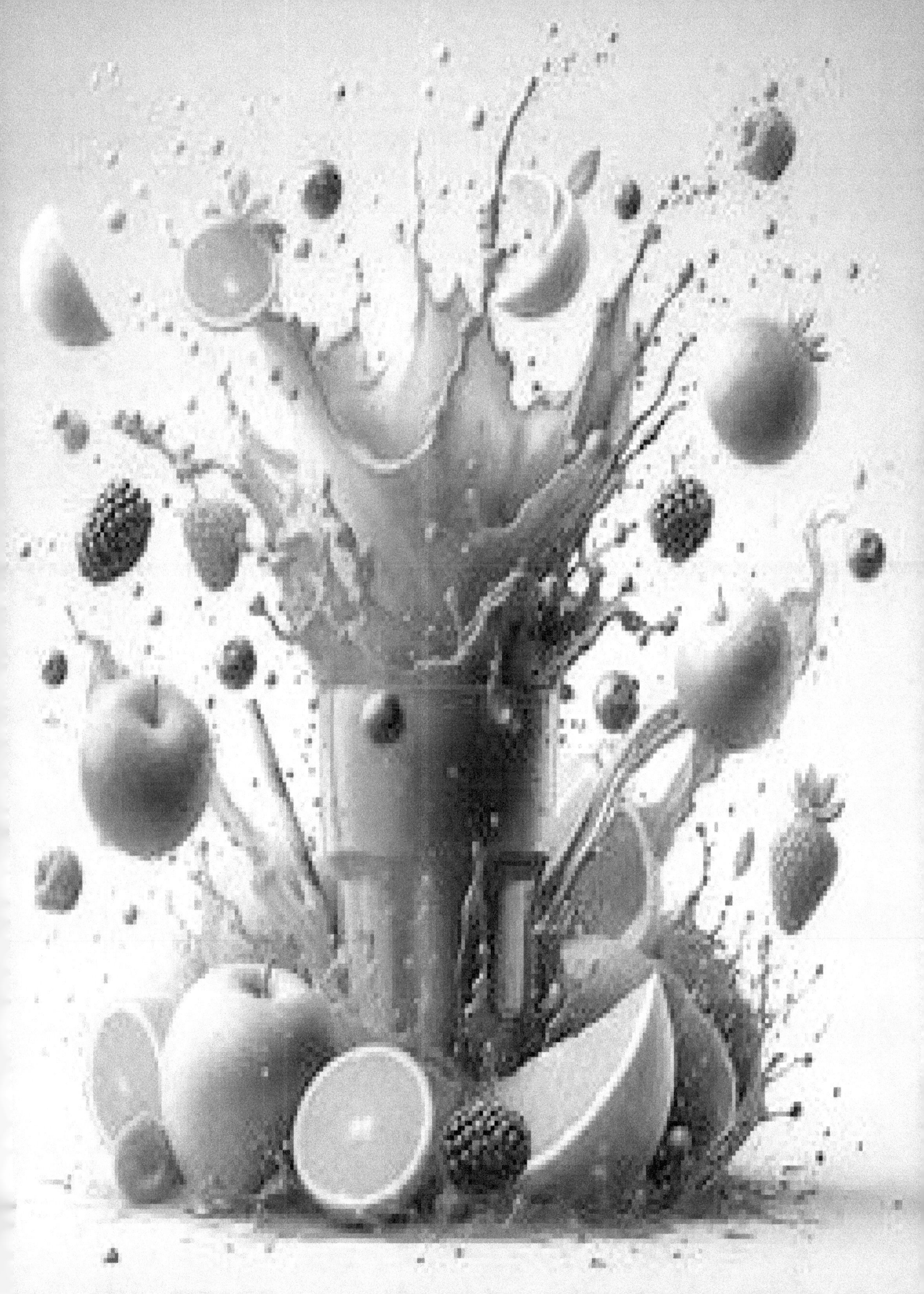